TRADITIONAL AND NOVEL RISK FACTORS IN ATHEROTHROMBOSIS

Edited by **Efraín Gaxiola**

Traditional and Novel Risk Factors in Atherothrombosis
Edited by Efraín Gaxiola

Published by InTech
Janeza Trdine 9, 51000 Rijeka, Croatia

Publishing Process Manager Anja Filipovic

Technical Editor Teodora Smiljanic

Cover Designer InTech Design Team

Additional hard copies can be obtained from orders@intechopen.com

Traditional and Novel Risk Factors in Atherothrombosis, Edited by Efraín Gaxiola
p. cm.
ISBN 978-953-51-0561-9

For EU product safety concerns:
IN TECH d.o.o., Prolaz Marije Krucifikse Kozulić 3, 51000 Rijeka, Croatia,
info@intechopen.com or visit our website at intechopen.com.

Meet the editor

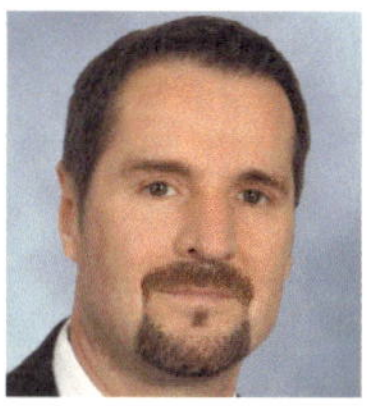

Dr Efraín Gaxiola is a Chief of Cardiac Catheterization Laboratory at Jardines Hospital de Especialidades in Guadalajara, México. He completed medical school at the Universidad Autónoma de Guadalajara and did his Internal Medicine training at Centro Médico La Raza in México City. After completing his cardiology fellowship training at Instituto Nacional de Cardiología "Ignacio Chávez" in México City, he was an Interventional Cardiology Fellow at the Univeristy of Florida in Gainesville, Florida. He is a former President of the Mexican Interventional Cardiology Society and the Latin American Interventional Cardiology Society. Dr. Gaxiola has been a member of TCT Faculty for more than 8 years and a member of the International Scientific Committee of the American College of Cardiology. He has published more than 80 manuscripts, mainly related to atherothrombosis, coronary artery disease, oral antiplatelet agents and has written more than 15 book chapters. His early research involved risk stratification and trials of antiplatelet and antithrombotic therapy in acute coronary syndromes.

Contents

Preface

Atherothrombosis has reached pandemic proportions worldwide. It is the underlying condition that results in events leading to myocardial infarction, ischemic stroke and vascular death. As such, it is the leading cause of death worldwide manifested mainly as cardiovascular/cerebrovascular death.

As the population of many countries becomes more aged, so the burden of atherothrombosis increases. The burden of atherothrombosis is felt in numerous ways: shortened life expectancy, increased morbidity and mortality and future risk of consequences in multiple systems.

Although therapeutic improvements and public health policies for risk factors control have brought about a reduction in atherothrombosis among the general population, this success has not been extended to some group populations as diabetics.

The complex and intimate relationship between atherothrombosis and traditional and novel risk factors is discussed in the following chapters of *Traditional and Novel Risk Factors in Atherothrombosis* – from basic science to clinical and therapeutic concerns. Beginning with pathology and pathophysiology of atherothrombosis, plaque rupture/disruption, this book continues with molecular, biochemical, inflammatory, cellular aspects and finally analyzes several aspects of clinical pharmacology.

This book is made up of seven chapters. In the first, Yamashita and Asada delineate the pathophysiologic mechanisms of plaque disruption and thrombus formation as critical steps for the onset of cardiovascular events, and that simultaneous activation of coagulation cascade and platelets play an important role in thrombus formation after plaque disruption. Next, Body, Slevin and McDowell discuss current methods for assessment of the presence, degree of severity and 'plaque composition' in patients with atherosclerosis, incuding current and novel imaging technology and measurement of circulating biomarkers of atherosclerosis. Subsequently, Watanabe and Koba clarify the roles of Serotonin in atherothrombosis and its related diseases, and how serotonin plays a crucial role in the formation of thrombosis and atherosclerotic lesions through 5-HT_{2A} receptors. Po-Hsun Huang analyzes the therapeutic use of endothelial progenitor cell in cardiovascular diseases. Yacoub, Hassan, Alaadine, Merhi, and Mourad discuss the role of CD40 Ligand and its receptors in atherothrombosis. They show that besides its pivotal role in humoral immunity, CD40L is now regarded as a key player to all major phases of atherothrombosis, a concept supported in part by the strong relationship between its circulating soluble levels and the occurrence of cardiovascular diseases. The last two chapters are dedicated to diagnostic and therapeutic issues. Shalia and Shah describe the current use of diagnostic biomarkers in ACS, as well as novel cardiac biomarkers of ACS. Sharma and Aronow talk about the optimal diagnosis and management of lower extremity peripheral arterial disease, detailing both the classical and modern therapeutic options.

I would like to pay tribute and express our appreciation to the distinguished and internationally renowned collaborators of this book for their outstanding contribution. Despite their many commitments and busy time schedules, all of them enthusiastically stated their acquiescence to cooperate. This book could not have become a reality were it not for their dedicated efforts.

Efraín Gaxiola, MD, FACC
Cardiology Chief
Jardínes Hospital de Especialidades
Guadalajara,
México

1

Pathology and Pathophysiology of Atherothrombosis: Virchow's Triad Revisited

Atsushi Yamashita and Yujiro Asada
University of Miyazaki, Japan

1. Introduction

In 1856, Rudolf Virchow published "Cellular pathology" based on macroscopic and microscopic observation of diseases, and described a triad of factors on thrombosis. The three components were vascular change, blood flow alteration, and abnormalities of blood constituents. Although Virchow originally referred to venous thrombosis, the theory can also be applied to arterial thrombosis, and it is considered that atherothrombus formation is regulated by the thrombogenicity of exposed plaque contents, local hemorheology, and blood factors. Thrombus formation on a disrupted atherosclerotic plaque is a critical event that leads to atherothrombosis. However, it does not always result in complete thrombotic occlusion with subsequent acute symptomatic events (Sato et al., 2009). Therefore, thrombus growth is also critical to the onset of clinical events. In spite of intensive investigation on the mechanisms of thrombus formation, little is known about the mechanisms involved in thrombogenesis or thrombus growth after plaque disruption, because thrombus is assessed with chemical or physical injury of "normal" arteries in most animal models of thrombosis.

Vascular change is an essential factor of atherothrombosis. Atherothrombosis is initiated by disruption of atherosclerotic plaque. The plaque disruption is morphologically characterized, however, the triggers of plaque disruption have not been completely understood. Tissue factor (TF) is an initiator of the coagulation cascade, is normally expressed in adventitia and variably in the media of normal artery (Drake et al., 1989). Because the atherosclerotic lesion expresses active TF, it is considered that TF in atherosclerotic lesion is a major determinant of vascular wall thrombogenicity (Owens & Mackman, 2010). Therefore, atherosclerotic lesions with TF expression are indispensable for studying atherothrombosis. To examine thrombus formation on TF-expressing atherosclerotic lesions, we established a rabbit model of atherothrombosis (Yamashita et al., 2003, 2009). This allowed us to investigate the "Virchow's triad" on atherothrombosis.

Blood flow is a key modulator of the development of atherosclerosis and thrombus formation. The areas of disturbed flow or low shear stress are susceptible for atherogenesis, whereas areas under steady flow and physiologically high shear stress are resistant to atherogenesis (Malek et al., 1999). The transcription of thrombogenic or anti-thrombogenic genes is also regulated by shear stress (Cunningham & Gotlieb, 2005). The blood flow can be altered by vascular stenosis, acute luminal change after plaque disruption, and micovascular constriction induced by distal embolism (Topol & Yadav, 2003). The blood flow alteration after plaque disruption may affect thrombus formation.

Blood circulates in the vessel as a liquid. This property suddenly changes after plaque disruption. The exposure of matrix proteins and TF induce platelet adhesion, aggregation and activation of coagulation cascade, resulted in platelet-fibrin thrombus formation. Clinical studies revealed increased platelet reactivity, coagulation factors, and reduced fibrinolytic activity in patients with atherothrombosis (Feinbloom & Bauer, 2005), and that risk factors for atherothrombosis can affect these blood factors (Lemkes et al., 2010, Rosito et al., 2004). In addition, recent evidences suggest that white blood cells can influence arterial thrombus formation. It seems that abnormalities on blood factors affect thrombus growth rather than initiation of thrombus formation.

This article focuses on pathology and pathophysiology of coronary atherothrombosis. Because mechanisms of atherothrombus formation are highly complicated, we separately discuss the "Virchow's triad" on atherothrombogenesis and thrombus growth.

2. Pathology of atherothrombosis

Traditionally, it is considered that arterial thrombi are mainly composed of aggregated platelets because of rapid blood flow condition, and the development of platelet-rich thrombi has been regarded as a cause of atherothrombosis. However, recent evidences indicate that atherothrombi are composed of aggregated platelets and fibrin, along erythrocytes and white blood cells, and constitutively immunopositive for GPIIb/IIIa (a platelet integrin), fibrin, glycophorin A (a membrane protein expressed on erythrocytes), von Willbrand factor (VWF, a blood adhesion molecule). And neutrophils are major white blood cells in coronary atherothrombus (Nishihira et al., 2010, Yamashita et al., 2006a). GPIIb/IIIa colocalized with VWF. TF was closely associated with fibrin (Yamashita et al., 2006a). The findings suggest that VWF and/or TF contribute thrombus growth and obstructive thrombus formation on atherosclerotic lesions, and that the enhanced platelet aggregation and fibrin formation indicate excess thrombin generation mediated by TF.

Overexpression of TF and its procoagulant activity have been found in human atherosclerotic plaque, and TF-expressing cells are identified as macrophages and smooth muscle cells (SMC) in the intima (Wilcox et al., 1989). The TF activity is more prominent in fatty streaks and atheromatous plaque than in the diffuse intimal thickening in aorta (Hatakeyama et al., 1997). Thus, atherosclerotic plaque has a potential to initiate coagulation cascade after plaque disruption, and TF in the plaque is thought to play an important role in thrombus formation after plaque disruption. Interestingly, TF pathway inhibitor (TFPI), a major down regulator of TF-factor VIIa (FVIIa) complex, is also upregulated in atherosclerotic lesions (Crawley et al., 2000). In addition to endothelial cells, macrophages, medial and intimal SMCs express TFPI. These evidence suggest that imbalance between TF and TFPI contribute to vascular wall thrombogenicity.

Two major patterns of plaque disruption are plaque rupture and plaque erosion (Figure 1). Plaque rupture is caused by fibrous cap disruption, allowing blood to come in contact with the thrombogenic necrotized core, resulting in thrombus formation. Ruptured plaque is characterized by disruption of thin fibrous caps, usually less than 65 μm in thickness, rich in macrophages and lymphocytes, and poor in SMCs (Virmani et al., 2000). Thus, the thinning of the fibrous cap is though to be a state vulnerable to rupture, the so-called thin-cap fibroatheroma (Kolodgie et al., 2001). However, the thin-cap fibroatheroma is not taken into account in the current American Heart Association classification of atherosclerosis (Stary et al., 1995). Plaque erosion is characterized by a denuded plaque surface and thrombus formation, and defined by the lack of surface disruption of the fibrous cap. Compared with plaque rupture, patients with plaque erosion are younger, no male predominance. Angiographycally, there is less narrowing and irregularity of the luminal surface in erosion. The morphologic characteristics include an abundance of SMCs and proteoglycan matrix, expecially versican and hyaluronan, and disruption of surface endothelium. Necrotic core is often absent. Plaque erosion contains relatively few macrophages and T cells compared with plaque rupture (Virmani et al., 2000). Thrombotic occlusion is less common with plaque erosion than plaque rupture, whereas microembolization in distal small vessels is more common with plaque erosion than plaque rupture (Schwartz et al., 2009). The proportions of fibrin and platelets differ in coronary thrombi on ruptured and eroded plaques. Thrombi on ruptured plaque are fibrin-rich, but those on eroded plaque are platelet-rich. TF and C reactive protein (CRP) are abundantly present in ruptured plaque, compared with eroded plaques (Sato et al., 2005). These distinct morphologic features suggest the different mechanisms in plaque rupture and erosion.

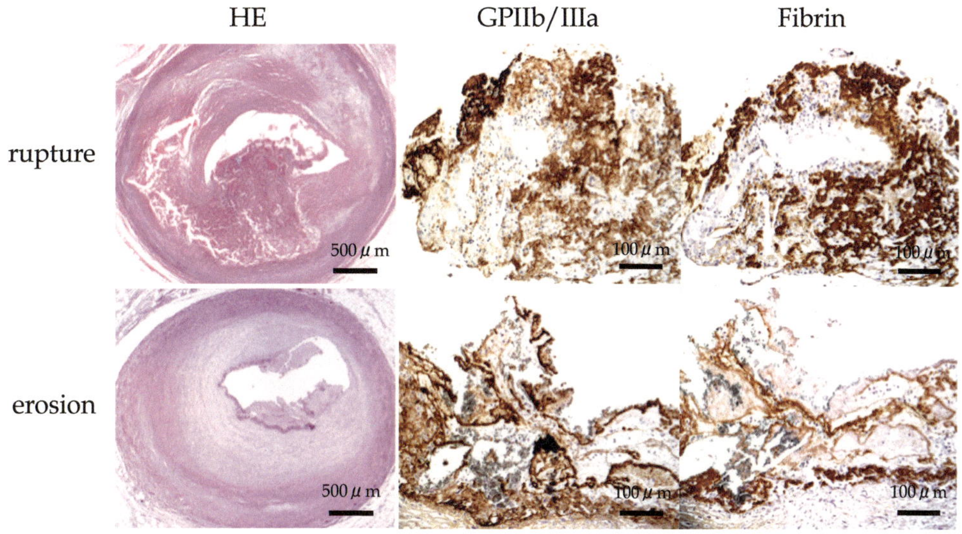

Fig. 1. Human coronary plaque rupture and erosion in patients with acute myocardial infarction.

Large necrotic core and disrupted thin fibrous cap is accompanied by thrombus formation in ruptured plaque. Eroded plaque has superficial injury of SMC-rich atherosclerotic lesion with thrombus formation. Both thrombi comprise platelets and fibrin. HE, Hematoxylin eosin stain (from Sato et al. 2005, with permission).

3. Pathology of asymptomatic atherothrombus

On the other hands, the disruption of atherosclerotic plaque does not always result in complete thrombotic occlusion with subsequent acute symptomatic events. The clinical studies using angioscopy have revealed that multiple plaque rupture is a frequent complication in patients with coronary atherothrombosis (Okada et al., 2011). Healed stages of plaque disruption are also occasionally observed in autopsy cases with or without coronary atherothrombosis (Burke et al., 2001). To evaluate the incidence and morphological characteristics of thrombi and plaque disruption in patients with non-cardiac death, Sato et al. (2009) examined 102 hearts from non-cardiac death autopsy cases and 19 from those who died of acute myocardical infarction (AMI). They found coronary thrombi in 16% of cases with non-cardiac death, and most of them developed on plaque erosion, and the thrombi were too small to affect coronary lumen (Figure 2, Table 1). The disrupted plaques in non-cardiac death case had smaller lipid areas, thicker fibrous caps, and more modest luminal narrowing than those in cases with AMI. A few autopsy studies have examined the incidence of coronary thrombus in non-cardiac death. Davies et al. (1989) and Arbustini et al. (1993) found 3 (4%) mural thrombi in 69, and 10 (7%) thrombi in 132 autopsy cases with non-cardiac death. The all coronary thrombi from non-cardiac death were associated with plaque erosion (Arbustini et al., 1993). Although the precise mechanisms of plaque erosion remain unknown, it is possible that the superficial erosive injury is a common mechanism of coronary thrombus formation. The results suggest that plaque disruption does not always result in complete thrombotic occlusion with subsequent acute symptomatic events, that thrombus growth is critical step for the onset of clinical events, and that at least the regional factors influence the size of coronary thrombus after plaque disruption.

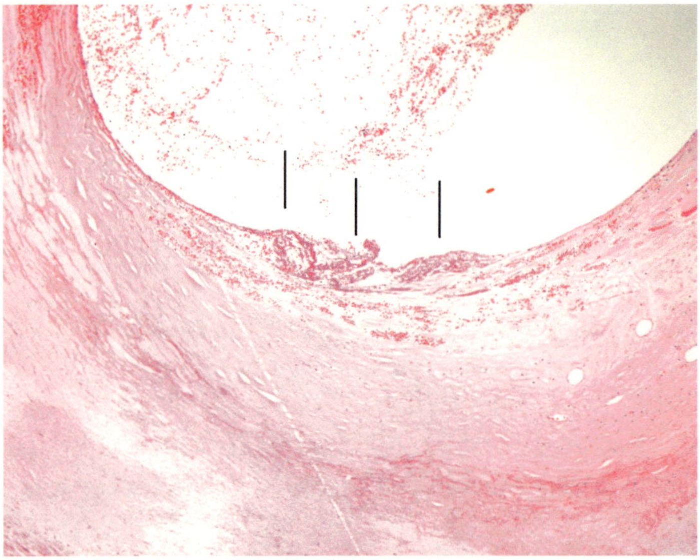

Fig. 2. Human coronary plaque erosion in patient with non-cardiac death.

	Non-cardiac death (n=102)	Acute myocardial infarction (n=19)	P value
Fresh thrombus	10 (10%)	14 (74%)	<0.001
erosion	7 (7%)	4 (21%)	0.07
rupture	3 (3%)	10 (53%)	<0.001
Old thrombus	6 (6%)	5 (26%)	<0.05

(From Sato et al. 2009, with permission)

Table 1. Incidence of thrombosis in non-cardiac death and acute myocardial infarction.

The atherosclerotic lesion shows superficial erosive injury with mural thrombus (arrows). The thrombus is too small to obstruct coronary lumen and induce symptomatic event (hematoxyline eosin stain, from Sato et al. 2009, with permission).

4. Pathophysiology of atherothrombosis

4.1 Triggers on plaque disruption

As described above, atherothrombosis is initiated by plaque rupture or plaque erosion. The plaque disruption is probably affected by vascular wall change and local blood flow. Our recent study revealed that disturbed blood flow could trigger plaque erosion in rabbit femoral artery with SMC-rich plaque. We separately discuss possible factors that affect plaque rupture or plaque erosion in atherosclerotic vessels.

4.1.1 Vascular change in plaque rupture

The thinning and disruption of fibrous cap by metalloproteases together with local rheological forces and emotional status is likely to be involved in plaque rupture. Accumulating evidence supports a key role for inflammation in the pathogenesis of plaque rupture. The inflammatory cells that appear quite numerous in rupture-prone atherosclerotic plaques can produce enzymes degrading the extracellular matrix of the fibrous cap. Macrophages in human atheroma overexpress interstitial collagenases and gelatinases, and elastolytic enzymes. Activated T lymphocytes and macrophages can secrete interferon γ (INF-γ), which inhibits collagen synthesis and induces apoptotic death of SMC (Shah, 2003). Moreover, INF-γ can induce interleukine (IL)-18, an accelerator of inflammation. IL-18 is colocalized with INF-γ in macrophage located at shoulder region, but not at necrotic core, and is associated with coronary thrombus formation in patients with ischemic heart disease (Nishihira et al., 2007). IL-10, an important anti-inflammatory cytokine, also is upregulated in macrophage in atherosclerotic lesion from patients with unstable angina compared with stable angina (Nishihira et al., 2006b). Heterogeneity of macrophages in atherosclerotic plaque could explain the paradoxical findings (Waldo et al., 2008). These evidences indicate that the imbalance of inflammatory pathway appear to participate in the destabilization of the plaque that triggers thrombosis in fibrous cap rupture.

Other possible trigger of plaque rupture is intraplaque hemorrhage. The frequency of previous hemorrhages is greater in coronary atherosclerotic lesions with late necrosis and thin fibrous cap than those lesions with early necrosis or intimal thickening (Kolodgie et al., 2003). Plaque hemorrhage is present in majority (>75%) of acute ruptures, and in 40% of fibrous cap and thin-fibrous cap atheromas. In addition, intraplaque hemorrhage is more frequently seen in patients with AMI compared to patients with healed myocardial infarction or non-cardiac death (Virmani et al., 2003). In coronary culprit lesions obtained by directional coronary atherectomy, intraplaque hemorrhage and iron deposition were more prominent in patients with unstable angina pectoris than with stable angina pectoris. The iron deposition correlated with oxidized low density lipoprotein and thioredoxin, an anti-oxidant protein, and was also associated with thrombus formation (Nishihira et al., 2008b). The pathological findings imply a possible relationship among intraplaque hemorrhage, oxidative stress, and plaque instability. However, the direct evidence that links intraplaque hemorrhage to plaque instability is still lacking.

4.1.2 Blood flow-induced mechanical stress on plaque rupture

Blood flow-induced mechanical stress is an essential factor of development of atherosclerosis and atherothrombosis. The low shear stress and oscillatory shear stress are both important stimuli for induction of atherosclerosis. Using a perivascular shear stress modifier in mice, Cheng et al. (2006) revealed that low shear stress induces larger lesions with vulnerable plaque phenotype (more lipids, more proteolytic enzymes, less SMCs, and less collagen) whereas vortices with oscillatory shear stress induce stable lesions. Chatzizisis et al. (2011) reported development of thin fibrous cap atheroma in coronary artery with low shear stress in pigs. In addition, the shear stress-induced changes in atherosclerotic plaque composition are modulated by chemokines. Inhibition of fractalkine, which is exclusively expressed in the low shear stress-induced atherosclerotic plaque, was reduced lipid and macrophage accumulation in the brachiocephalic arteries in mice (Cheng et al., 2007). Therefore, lower shear stress can induce atherosclerotic lesion prone to plaque rupture. Although it is well recognized that a mechanical stress triggers the disruption of fibrous cap, it remains unclear which factor is mainly responsible for the disruption of the thin fibrous cap. A variety of mechanical factors have been postulated to play a role in plaque rupture, including hemodynamic shear stress, turbulent pressure fluctuation (Loree et al., 1991), sudden increases in intraluminal pressure (Muller et al., 1989), and tensile stress concentration within the wall of the lesion. To investigate the relationship between shear stress distribution and coronary plaque rupture, Fukumoto et al. (2008) analyzed 3-dimmensional intravascular ultrasound images in patients with acute coronary thrombosis by a program for calculating the fluid dynamics. The ruptured sites were located in the proximal or top portion of the plaques, and the localized high shear stress is frequently correlated with the rupture sites. This finding is inconsistent with role of low shear stress on atherogenesis. It is possible that the process of initiating plaque rupture is quite different form that of atherogenesis. On the other hand, an excessive concentration of tensile stress within the plaque may be one of the triggers of plaque rupture. When the tensile stress becomes greater than the fragility of the fibrous cap, a plaque disruption may be initiated. The tensile stress is increased by development of a lipid core, thinning of the fibrous cap (Loree et al., 1992). Cheng et al. (1993) analyzed the distribution of circumferential stress in human coronary arteries. The maximum circumferential stress in ruptured plaques was significantly higher than that in stable plaques, although plaque rupture does not always occur at the region of highest stress. These results suggest that a mechanical factor that triggers plaque rupture differ in each case and lesion.

4.1.3 Disturbed blood flow on plaque erosion

Although it has been postulated that erosions result from coronary vasospasm of SMC-rich plaque, the mechanisms of plaque erosion are poorly understood. Approximately 80% thrombi of plaque erosion are nonocclusive in spite of sudden coronary death (Virmani et al., 2000). Platelet rich emboli are found in 74% of patients dying suddenly with plaque erosion compared with plaque rupture (40%). Because activated platelets release vasoconstrictive agents, such as 5-hydroxytriptamine (5-HT, serotonin) and thromboxane A2, these emboli might increase peripheral resistance leading to alteration of coronary blood flow. 5-HT can induce vasoconstriction and reduce coronary blood flow in human atherosclerotic vessels but not in normal arteries (Golino et al., 1991).

Experimental aortic stenosis can induce acute endothelial change or damage of the normal aorta (Fry, 1968). Therefore, hemodynamic force, particularly disturbed blood flow induced by stenosis or vasoconstriction, could be a crucial factor in generating surface vascular damage and thrombosis. To address the relation between disturbed blood flow and plaque erosion, we investigated the pathological change after acute luminal narrowing in SMC-rich plaque in rabbit. The SMC-rich plaque was induced by a balloon injury of rabbit femoral artery, and expressed TF as human atherosclerotic plaques. Actually, the disturbed blood by acute vascular narrowing induced superficial erosive injury to the SMC-rich plaque at post stenotic regions in rabbit femoral arteries. Figure 3 shows microscopic images of the longitudinal section of the neointima at the post- stenotic region 15 min after vascular narrowing. The endothelial cells and SMCs at this region were broadly detached with time, and associated with platelet adhesion to the sub-endothelium. Apoptosis of endothelial cells

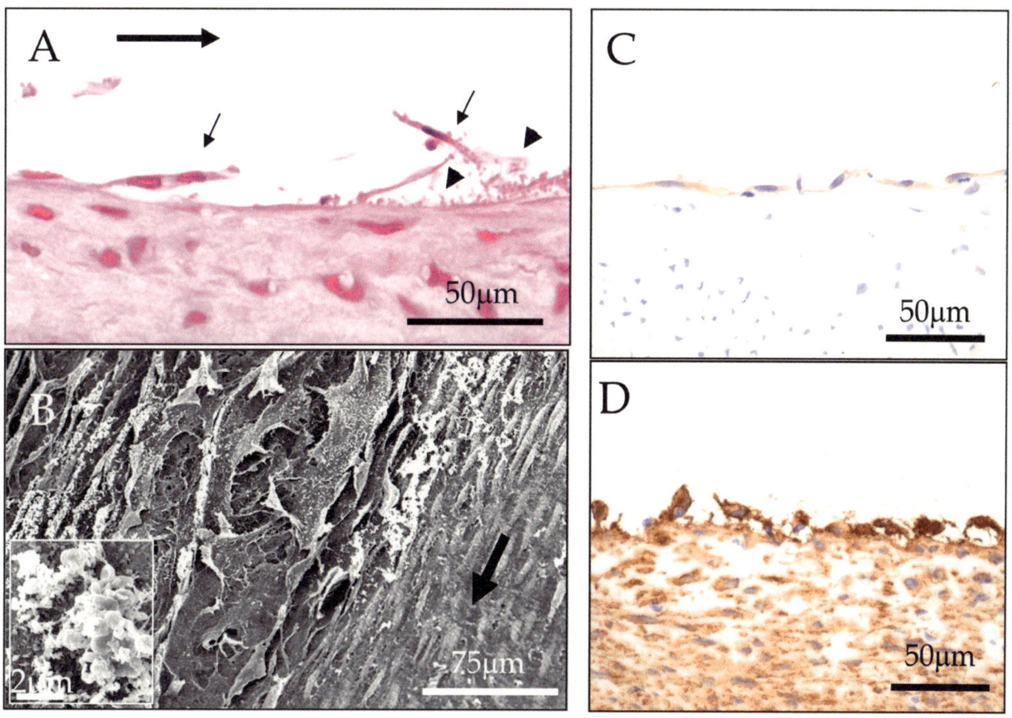

Fig. 3. Representative images of superficial erosive injury of SMC-rich plaque and thrombus formation at the post-stenotic region.
SMC-rich plaque 15 min after vascular narrowing shows endothelial detachement (small arrows) accompanies platelet adhesion (arrow heads) at 1mm form vascular narrowing (A, hematoxyline eosin stain). Detachment of endothelial cells and exposure of subendothelial matrix is accompanied by platelet aggregation on the left side, and residual endothelial cell layer is present on right side (inset, high magnification of aggregated platelets) (B. scanning electron microscopy). Immunohistochemistry for VWF (C, a marker of endothelium) or smooth muscle actin (D, a marker of SMC) confirm detachment of endothelial cells and SMCs at post stenotic region (from Sumi et al. 2010, with permission).

and superficial SMCs was also observed at the post- stenotic region within 15 minutes (Sumi et al., 2010). The vascular narrowing induced large mural thrombi which composed of platelets and fibrin, as human plaque erosion. Thus, disturbed blood flow can induce superficial erosive injury to SMC-rich plaque and thrombus formation at post stenotic region. Computational fluid simulation analysis indicated that oscillatory shear stress contributes to the development of the erosive damage to the plaque (Sumi et al., 2010). Although direct clinical evidence has not yet supported the notion that coronary artery vasospasm plays a role in plaque erosion, the superficial erosive injury of SMC-rich plaque by disturbed blood flow is similar to those of human plaque erosion (Sato et al., 2005). And, platelet and blood coagulation in coronary circulation are activated after vasospastic angina (Miyamoto et al. 2001, Oshima et al., 1990). Therefore, these evidence suggest that an acute-onset disturbed blood flow due to vasoconstriction could trigger plaque erosion. Hemodynamic factors could play an important role in development of plaque erosion.

4.2 Virchow's triads on thrombus growth

As described above, plaque disruption does not always result in complete thrombotic occlusion. Thrombus growth is considered critical to the onset of clinical events. Although thrombus formation is regulated by the vascular wall thrombogenicity, local blood flow, and blood contents, their contribution to thrombus growth has not been clearly defined. We separately discuss three factors that affect thrombus growth in atherosclerotic vessels.

4.2.1 Vascular factors on thrombus growth

Most fundamental difference between normal artery and atherosclerotic artery is presence of abundant active TF in atherosclerotic lesions (Hatakeyama et al., 1997, Wilcox et al., 1989). It seems that vascular wall TF contribute to thrombus size/propagation on atherosclerotic lesions. However, recent studies indicate that a small amount of TF is detectable in the blood and is capable of supporting clot formation in vitro. Plasma TF levels are elevated in patients with unstable angina and AMI and correlate with adverse outcomes (Mackman, 2004). Therefore, it is still controversial whether vascular wall and/or blood-derived TF support thrombus propagation. Hematopoietic cell-derived, TF-positive microparticles contributed to laser injury-induced thrombosis in the microvasculature of mouse cremaster muscle (Chou et al. 2004). In contrast, vascular smooth muscle-derived TF contributed to $FeCl_3$ induced thrombosis in mouse carotid artery (Wang et al., 2009). We investigated whether plaque and/or blood TF contribute to thrombus formation in rabbit femoral artery with or without atherosclerotic lesions. The atherosclerotic lesions in rabbit femoral arteries were induced by a 0.5% cholesterol diet and balloon injury, and showed TF expression and increased procoagulant activity compared with normal femoral arteries (Figure 4). Balloon injury of the atherosclerotic plaque induced thrombin-dependent large platelet-fibrin thrombi. In contrast, balloon injury of normal femoral artery induced thrombin-independent small platelet thrombi (Figure 5). Moreover, whole blood coagulation in the rabbits was not affected by blood TF inhibition with a TF antibody even in hyperlipidemic condition (Yamashita et al., 2009). Therefore, at least, atherosclerotic plaque-derived TF might contribute to activation of intravascular coagulation cascade and thrombus size/propagation on atherosclerotic lesions.

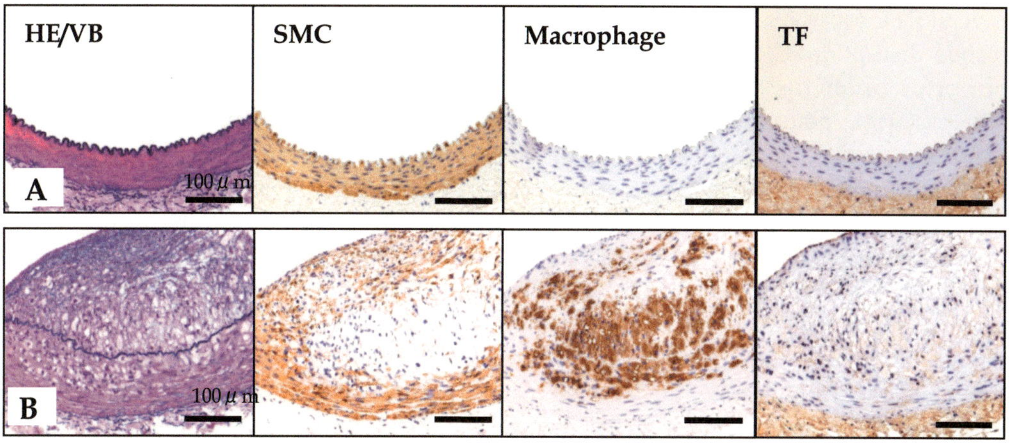

Fig. 4. Histological images of rabbit femoral arteries.
Representative immunohistochemical microphotographs of normal (A) and balloon-injured femoral artery at 3 weeks after injury under 0.5% cholesterol diet (B). Atherosclerotic lesion composed of SMCs and macrophages develops in injured artery. TF expression is present in the lesion and adventitia of both arteries. HE/VB, hematoxyline eosin/Victoria blue stain (From Yamashita et al. 2009, with permission).

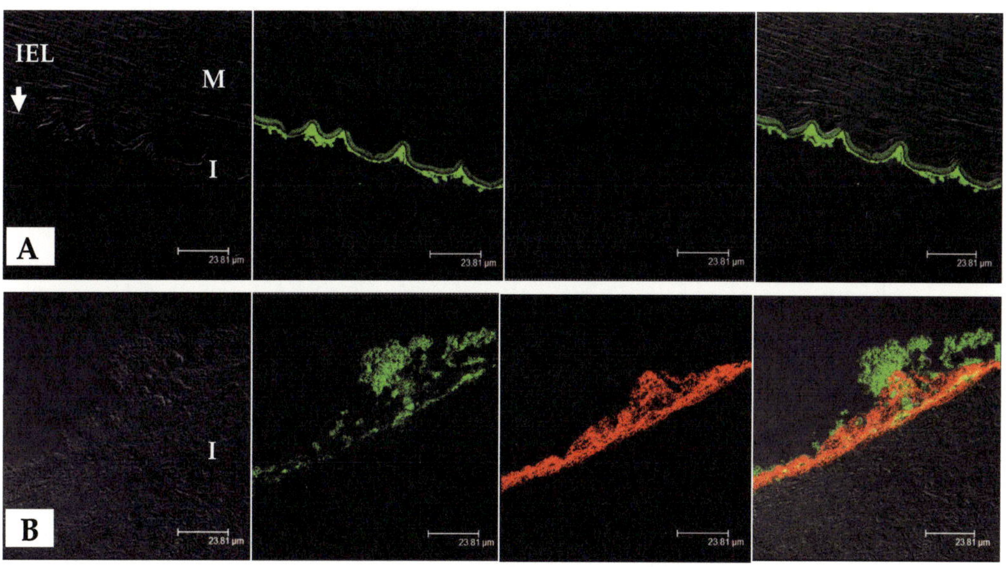

Fig. 5. Immunofluorescence images of thrombus on rabbit femoral artery.
Representative immunofluorescent microphotographs of thrombi 15 minutes after balloon injury of normal femoral artery and of atherosclerotic plaque under 0.5% cholesterol diet. Rows show differential interference contrast images, images stained with fluorescein isothiocyanate-labeled GPIIb/IIIa (green), Cy3-labeled fibrin (red), and merged immunofluorescent images. Areas with colocalized factors are stained yellow. The thrombi on normal intima is composed of small aggregated platelet (A), while the thrombi on atherosclerotic plaque is large, and composed of platelet and fibrin (B). I, intima; M, media; IEL, internal elastic lamina. (From Yamashita et al. 2009, with permission).

Several factors can influence TF expression in plaques and atherothrombus formation after plaque disruption. CRP is an inflammatory acute-phase reactant that has emerged as a powerful predictor of cardiovascular disease (Ridker, 2007). CRP is localized in atherosclerotic plaques and is more in thrombotic plaques than non-thrombotic ones (Ishikawa et al., 2003, Sun et al., 2005). The findings imply that CRP is implicated in atherothrombogenesis. To address this issue, CRP-transgenic rabbits were generated, because as human CRP, CRP in rabbits but not in mice works as an acute-phase reactant during inflammation (Koike et al., 2009). In the rabbits, CRP was overexpressed in livers and circulated in blood and deposited in the both SMC-rich and macrophage-rich atherosclerotic lesions. The thrombus size on SMC-rich plaque or macrophage-rich plaque after balloon injury was significantly increased in CRP-transgenic rabbits as compared with wild non-transgenic rabbits (Figure 6). TF expression and its acivity in the plaques were significantly increased in CRP-transgenic rabbits. The degree of CRP deposition correlated with TF expression in plaques and thrombus size on injured plaques (Matsuda et al., 2011). On the

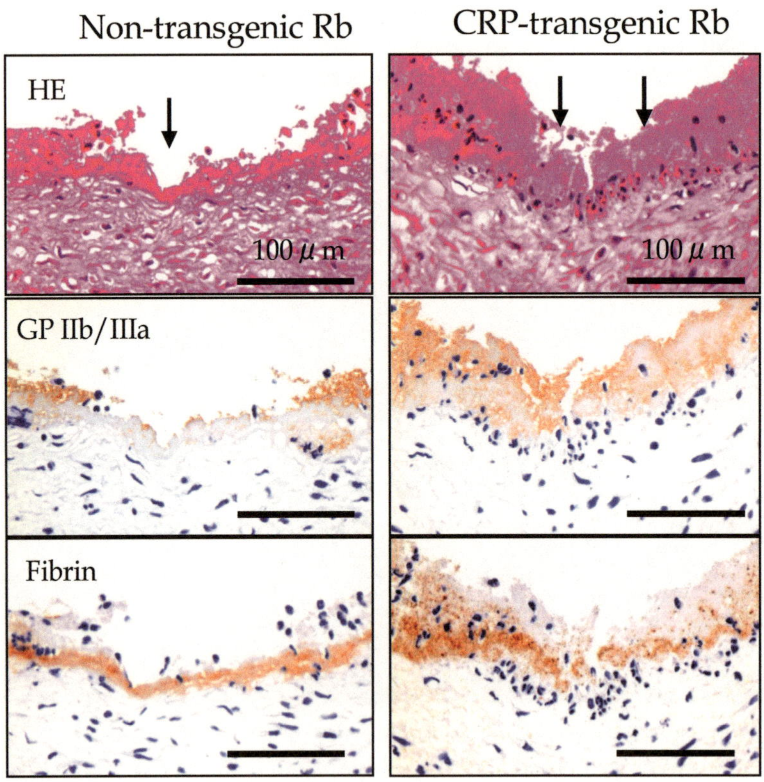

Fig. 6. Thrombus formation on SMC-rich plaque in CRP-transgenic or non-transgenic rabbit femoral artery.
The images show thrombus formation on SMC-rich plaque (arrows) 15 min after balloon injury of rabbit femoral arteries. The thrombus size is increased in CRP-transgenic rabbits as compared with non-transgenic rabbit. Immunopositive areas for GPIIb/IIIa and fibrin also increase in CRP-transgenic rabbit (from Matsuda et al. 2011, with permission).

other hand, the CRP overexpression did not enhance atherosclerosis induced by hyperchoresterol diets (Koike et al., 2009). CRP localized in atherosclerotic plaques might enhance vascular wall thrombogenicity and thrombus formation after plaque disruption rather than atherogenesis.

4.2.2 Altered blood flow on thrombus growth

Blood flow is a key modulator of thrombus growth. Clinical studies revealed an alteration of coronary blood flow in patients with ischemic heart diseases. Marzilli et al. (2000) reported an approximate 80% reduction in coronary blood flow during ischemia in patients with unstable angina. An autopsy study reported that intramyocardial microemboli were frequently present in sudden coronary death patients (Schwartz et al. 2009). Distal microvascular embolism and/or vasoconstriction could affect blood flow alteration and thrombus formation and growth at the culprit lesions (Erbel & Heusch, 2000). To assess the issue, we examined the effects of the blood flow reduction to thrombus formation in our animal model. Blood flow reduction (>75%) promoted the growth of thrombus, a mixture of platelets and fibrin, on atherosclerotic lesion, which grew to occlusive one. The flow reduction also induced thrombus formation on normal arteries, but the thrombi were very small and composed only of platelets (Yamashita et al. 2004). Therefore, blood flow reduction associated with increased vascular wall thrombogenecity is considered to contribute thrombus growth. We also demonstrated an important role of 5-HT_{2A} receptor on platelets and SMCs in this process via platelet aggregation and thrombogenic vasoconstriction (Nishihira et al., 2006a, 2008a).

In addition to distal vascular resistance, disturbed blood flow by acute vascular narrowing promotes thrombus growth at post stenotic regions. As described above, vascular narrowing of rabbit femoral artery induced superficial erosive injury to SMC-rich plaque at post stenotic regions. The thrombi consisted of a mixture of aggregated platelets and a considerable amount of fibrin. The whole blood hemostatic parameters in the rabbits was not changed after vascular narrowing or anti-rabbit TF antibody treatment, which evidence indicates that TF derived from eroded plaque rather than circulating TF plays an important role in fibrin generation and thrombus growth (Sumi et al. 2010).

The rheological effect on thrombus growth may be partly explained by a shear gradient-dependent platelet aggregation mechanism. Using in vitro and in vivo stenotic microvessels and imaging systems, Nesbitt et al. (2009) revealed a shear gradient-dependent platelet aggregation process which is preceded by soluble agonist-dependent aggregation. Shear microgradient at post stenosis region or down stream face of thrombi induced stable platelets aggregates, and the shear microgradients directly influenced the platelet aggregation size. This process required ligand binding to integrin $\alpha IIb\beta 3$, transient Ca^{2+} flux, but did not required global platelet shape change or soluble agonists. The findings suggest that platelets principally use a biomechanical platelet aggregation mechanism in early phase of platelet adhesion and aggregation. Vessel and/or thrombus geometry itself may promote thrombus formation.

4.2.3 Blood factors on thrombus growth

As described above, platelet is a major cellular component in coronary thrombus, and platelets play an important role in growing phase of thrombus formation, as well as initial phase of thrombus formation. Adhesion molecules and its receptors on platelets are essential for thrombus formation, because these molecules support platelet tethering, firm adhesion, aggregation and platelet recruitment to thrombus surface. VWF is a large, multimeric, plasma protein that undergoes a conformational change when bound to matrix under permit its binding to GPIbα. Recent studies in vitro and in vivo showed that platelet recruitment on thrombus surface was primary mediated by VWF and GPIbα on flowing platelets (Bergmeier et al. 2006, Kulkuni et al. 2000). We demonstrated that a large amount of VWF was localized in coronary thrombi in patients with AMI (Nishihira et al., 2010, Yamashita et al., 2006a), and that monoclonal antibody against VWF A1 domain, which interacts platelet GPIbα, significantly suppressed formation of platelet-fibrin thrombi and completely inhibited occlusive thrombus formation in rabbit atherosclerotic lesions (Yamashita et al., 2003, 2004). These findings indicated a crucial role of VWF in thrombus growth via platelet recruitment. The multimer size of VWF can affect thrombus size and is regulated by a plasma protease, a disintegrin and metalloprotease with a thrombospondin type 1 motif 13 (ADAMTS-13). A deficiency of ADAMTS-13 activity causes an increased level of circulating ultralarge VWF multimers, and correlates with the onset of the general thrombotic disease, thrombotic thrombocytopenic purpura (TTP). A clinical evidence suggested dysregulation of VWF multimer size in AMI patient. The ratio of VWF/ADAMTS-13 antigen was higher in patients with AMI than in those with stable angina pectris, and there was a inverse correlation between plasma VWF antigen and ADAMTS-13 activity in AMI patients (Kaikita et al. 2006). The ADAMTS-13 closely localized with VWF in fresh coronary thrombi from AMI patients (Moriguchi-Goto et al., 2009). A reducing ADAMTS-13 activity by monoclonal antibody against distintegrin-like domain enhanced platelet thrombus growth on immobilized type I collagen at a high shear rate ($1500S^{-1}$) and platelet-fibrin thrombus formation on injured atherosclerotic lesion of rabbit femoral arteries (Moriguchi-Goto et al., 2009). The study also showed cleavage of large sized VWF multimer during platelet thrombus formation under a high shear rate. The VWF-cleaving site by ADAMTS-13 localized on the surface of platelet thrombus, and the ADAMTS-13 activity was shear dependent manner (Shida et al. 2008). Thus, ADAMTS-13 may work at the site of ongoing thrombus generation and limit thrombus growth.

The recent studies in vitro showed various blood cells, not only monocytes but also neutrophils, eosinophils, and even if platelets, can synthesize TF. Although there is much on debate on the TF expression in blood cells, it is likely that monocytes are the only blood cells that synthesize and express TF (Østerud, 2010). A related topic is contribution of microparticles (MPs) to thrombus formation. MPs are small fragments of membrane-bound cytoplasm that are shed from the surface of an activated or apoptotic cells (Blann et al. 2009). The procoagulant activity of MPs is increased with the exposure of phosphatidylserine and the presence of TF. In fact, MPs have significantly elevated in acute coronary syndrome and ischemic strokes (Geiser et al. 1998, Singh et al. 1995). However, it is still unclear whether the elevated levels of MPs are a cause or consequence of atherothrombosis. Moreover, our animal studies did not support the role of blood-derived TF in atherothrombus formation as described above. Future studies are required to clarify contribution of blood derived TF and/or MPs to thrombus propagation on atherosclerotic lesions.

Among the white blood cells, neutrophils are mostly found in coronary thrombus in patients with AMI, and CD34 positive leukocytes are also found in the thrombus (Nishihira et al., 2010). Recent evidences revealed neutrophils and endothelial progenitor cells influence thrombus growth. Neutrophils can positively or negatively affect thrombus formation by degradation of coagulation or fibrinolysis factors and promoting platelet function (Kornecki et al., 1988, Moir et al., 2002). Inhibition of interaction between p-selectin and p-selectin glycoprotein ligand 1 reduced fibrin formation in vivo (Palabrica et al., 1992). These adhesion molecules have been implicated in recruitment of leukocytes and leukocyte MPs to thrombi (Vandendries et al., 2004). To reveal the neutrophil-mediated procoagulant mechanisms, Massberg et al. (2010) investigated thrombus formation using neutrophil elastase and cathepsin G deficient mice. Proteolysis of TFPI by these proteases enhanced fibrin and thrombus formation after $FeCl_3$-induced vessel injury. In addition, activated platelets by collagen accelerated nucleosome externalization by neutrophils. The neutrophil-derived externalized nucleosomes can form neutrophil extracellular traps that provide a scaffold for platelets and red blood cells and histone 3/4 can induce platelet aggregation (Fuchs et al., 2010). On the other hands, neutrophil elastase has fibriolytic potential, and there is significant correlation between neutrophil elastase-digested fibrin and leukocyte content in human atherothrombi (Rábai et al., 2010). Zeng et al. (2002) investigated contribution of polymorphonuclear leukocytes (PMNs) to fibrinolysis in vivo using plasminogen deficient mice. The PMNs accumulated within the thrombi by 6 hours after $FeCl_3$-induced vessel injury and peaked at 24 hours. There were no significant differences between the PMNs from plasminogen deficient mice and wild type mice within the 6 hour after thrombus formation, whereas there was significant greater retention of PMNs within the thrombus over 24 hours after thrombus formation. PMNs from both mice showed fibrinolytic activity, but the degradation products were a distinct pattern. Therefore, it is possible that neutrophils works as positive or negative regulator of early or late phase of thrombus formation, respectively.

Endothelial progenitor cells (EPC) contributes to angiogenesis and wound healing (Asahara et al., 1997), and the number of EPCs in blood is associated with cardiovascular risk (Hill et al., 2003). The mechanisms that regulate mobilization, migration, and differentiation of EPCs and their homing to sites of vascular injury are complex and involve several mediators and receptors, such as P-selectin glycoprotein ligand-1, CXC chemokine, and integrins (Chavakis et al., 2005, Massberg et al., 2006). Interaction of thrombus contents and EPCs influences their mobilization and differentiation to mature endothelial cells during vascular injury (de Boer HC et al., 2006). Abou-Saleh et al. (2009) reported that human peripheral blood mononuclear cell derived EPCs bound platelets via p-selectin and inhibit platelet activation, aggregation, and adhesion to collagen in vitro, and that injection of these EPCs reduced thrombus formation after $FeCl_3$-induced vessel injury of mouse carotid arteries.

Other possible mechanism contributing thrombus propagation in vivo is intrinsic coagulation pathway. The intrinsic coagulation pathway is initiated when coagulation factor XII (FXII) comes into contact with negatively charged surfaces in a reaction involving the plasma proteins, high molecular mass kininogen and plasma kallikrein. Factor XI (FXI) is activated by activated FXII, thrombin, and activated XI. Feedback activation of FXI by thrombin promotes further thrombin generation in vitro (Gailani & Broze, 1991). FXI was present in platelet-fibrin thrombus induced balloon injury of atherosclerotic lesion in rabbits, and anti-FXI antibody reduced thrombus growth without prolonging bleeding (Yamashita et al., 2006b). FXI plays an important role in thrombus growth via further thrombin generation. On the other hand, there are conflicts of evidence that FXII supports arterial thrombus growth. FXII deficient mice were resistant to thrombotic occlusion after $FeCl_3$ induced vessel injury of carotid arteries (Cheng Q et al., 2010). However, a clinical study demonstrated an inverse relationship between FXII level and risk of myocardial infarction (Doggen et al., 2006). Moreover, inhibition of FXII did not change platelet aggregation and fibrin formation on atherosclerotic plaque surface under flow in vitro. The effect of FXII on coagulation became obvious only absence of TF (Reininger et al., 2010).

5. Conclusion

More than 150 years ago, Virchow described the mechanims of thrombus formation. It has still remained as a fundamental theory of thrombus formation. To date, pathological and experimental studies have clarified the mechanisms of atherothrombus formation. The thrombus formation is initiated by plaque rupture and plaque erosion. Among the Virchow's triad, vascular and rheological factors are responsible for plaque rupture. Disruption of thin fibrous cap atheroma triggers plaque rupture. On the other hand, disturbed blood by acute luminal change can trigger plaque erosion to SMC-rich plaque. Pathological findings of human atherothrombosis suggest that thrombus growth rather than plaque disruption is a critical step for the onset of cardiovascular events, and that simultaneous activation of coagulation cascade and platelets play an important role in thrombus formation after plaque disruption. All three factors contribute to atherothrombus growth. Our rabbit model of atherothrombosis revealed that excess thrombin generation mediated by plaque TF contribute to large plate-fibrin thrombus formation on atherosclerotic lesion, and that disturbed flow condition after plaque disruption promote thrombus growth. Recent evidence suggests that leukocytes influence arterial thrombus formation as well as platelet and coagulation/fibrinolysis factors. Differences between hemostasis and thrombus growth may shed light on a novel anti-atherothrombogic drug with a wide safety margin.

6. Acknowledgement

The work is supported in part by Grants-in-Aid for Scientific Research in Japan (No.23790410), Mitsubishi Pharma Research Foundation, and Integrated Research Project for Human and Veterinary Medicine.

7. References

Abou-Saleh, H., Yacoub, D., Théorêt, JF., Gillis, MA., Neagoe, PE., Labarthe, B., Théroux, P., Sirois, MG., Tabrizian, M., Thorin, E., & Merhi, Y. (2009). Endothelial progenitor cells bind and inhibit platelet function and thrombus formation. *Circulation*, Vol.120, No.22, pp.2230-2239.

Arbustini, E., Grasso, M., Diegoli, M., Morbini, P., Aguzzi, A., Fasani, R., & Specchia, G. (1993). Coronary thrombosis in non-cardiac death. *Coron Artery Dis*, Vol.4, No.9, pp.751-759.

Asahara, T., Murohara, T., Sullivan, A., Silver, M., van der Zee, R., Li, T., Witzenbichler, B., Schatteman, G., & Isner, JM. (1997). Isolation of putative progenitor endothelial cells for angiogenesis. *Science*. Vol.275, No.5302, pp.964-967.

Bergmeier, W., Piffath, CL., Goerge, T., Cifuni, SM., Ruggeri, ZM., Ware, J., & Wagner, DD. (2006). The role of platelet adhesion receptor GPIbalpha far exceeds that of its main ligand, von Willebrand factor, in arterial thrombosis. *Proc Natl Acad Sci U S A*. Vol.103, No.45, pp.16900-16905.

Blann, A., Shantsila, E., & Shantsila, A. (2009). Microparticles and arterial disease. *Semin Thromb Hemost*. Vol.35, No.5, pp.488-496.

Burke, AP., Kolodgie, FD., Farb, A., Weber, DK., Malcom, GT., Smialek J, & Virmani R. (2001). Healed plaque ruptures and sudden coronary death: evidence that subclinical rupture has a role in plaque progression. *Circulation*, Vol.103, No.7, pp.934-940.

Chatzizisis, YS., Baker, AB., Sukhova, GK., Koskinas, KC., Papafaklis, MI., Beigel, R., Jonas, M., Coskun, AU., Stone, BV., Maynard, C., Shi, GP., Libby, P., Feldman, CL., Edelman, ER., & Stone, PH. (2011). Augmented expression and activity of extracellular matrix-degrading enzymes in regions of low endothelial shear stress colocalize with coronary atheromata with thin fibrous caps in pigs. *Circulation*, Vol.123, No.6, pp.621-630.

Chavakis, E., Aicher, A., Heeschen, C., Sasaki, K., Kaiser, R., El Makhfi, N., Urbich, C., Peters, T., Scharffetter-Kochanek, K., Zeiher, AM., Chavakis, T., & Dimmeler, S. (2005). Role of beta2-integrins for homing and neovascularization capacity of endothelial progenitor cells. *J Exp Med*, Vol.201, No.1, pp.63-72Chou, J., Mackman, N., Merrill-Skoloff, G., Pedersen, B., Furie, BC., & Furie, B. (2004). Hematopoietic cell-derived microparticle tissue factor contributes to fibrin formation during thrombus propagation. *Blood*, Vol.104, No.10, pp.3190-3197.

Cheng, C., Tempel, D., van Haperen, R., van der Baan, A., Grosveld, F., Daemen, MJ., Krams, R., & de Crom, R. (2006). Atherosclerotic lesion size and vulnerability are determined by patterns of fluid shear stress. *Circulation*, Vol.113, No.23, pp.2744-2753.

Cheng, C., Tempel, D., van Haperen, R., de Boer, HC., Segers, D., Huisman, M., van Zonneveld, AJ., Leenen, PJ., van der Steen, A., Serruys, PW., de Crom, R., & Krams, R. (2007). Shear stress-induced changes in atherosclerotic plaque composition are modulated by chemokines. *J Clin Invest*, Vol.117, No.3, pp.616-626.

Cheng, GC., Loree, HM., Kamm, RD., Fishbein, MC., & Lee, RT. (1993). Distribution of circumferential stress in ruptured and stable atherosclerotic lesions. A structural analysis with histopathological correlation. *Circulation*, Vol.87, No.4, pp.1179-1187.

Cheng, Q., Tucker, EI., Pine, MS., Sisler, I., Matafonov, A., Sun, MF., White-Adams, TC., Smith, SA., Hanson, SR., McCarty, OJ., Renné, T., Gruber, A., & Gailani, D. (2010). A role for factor XIIa-mediated factor XI activation in thrombus formation in vivo. *Blood*. Vol.116, No.19, pp.3981-3989.

Chou, J., Mackman, N., Merrill-Skoloff, G., Pedersen, B., Furie, BC., & Furie, B. (2004). Hematopoietic cell-derived microparticle tissue factor contributes to fibrin formation during thrombus propagation. *Blood*, Vol.104, No.10, pp.3190-3197.

Crawley, J., Lupu, F., Westmuckett, AD., Severs, NJ., Kakkar, VV., & Lupu, C. (2000). Expression, localization, and activity of tissue factor pathway inhibitor in normal and atherosclerotic human vessels. *Arterioscler Thromb Vasc Biol*, Vol.20, No.5, pp.1362-1373.

Cunningham, KS., & Gotlieb, AI. (2005). The role of shear stress in the pathogenesis of atherosclerosis. *Lab Invest*, Vol.85, No.1, pp.9-23.

Davies, MJ., Bland, JM., Hangartner, JR., Angelini, A., & Thomas, AC. (1989). Factors influencing the presence or absence of acute coronary artery thrombi in sudden ischaemic death. *Eur Heart J*, Vol.10, No.3, pp.203-208.

Doggen, CJ., Rosendaal, FR., & Meijers, JC. (2006). Levels of intrinsic coagulation factors and the risk of myocardial infarction among men: Opposite and synergistic effects of factors XI and XII. *Blood*, Vol.108, No.13, pp.4045-4051.

Drake, TA., Morrissey, JH., & Edgington, TS. (1989). Selective cellular expression of tissue factor in human: Implications for disorders of hemostasis and thrombosis. *Am J Pathol,* Vol.134, No.5, pp.1087-1097

de Boer, HC., Verseyden, C., Ulfman, LH., Zwaginga, JJ., Bot, I., Biessen, EA., Rabelink, TJ., & van Zonneveld, AJ. (2006). Fibrin and activated platelets cooperatively guide stem cells to a vascular injury and promote differentiation towards an endothelial cell phenotype. *Arterioscler Thromb Vasc Biol,* Vol.26, No.7, pp.1653-1659.

Erbel, R., & Heusch, G. (2000). Coronary microembolization. *J Am Coll Cardiol,* Vol.36, No.1, pp.22-24.

Feinbloom D, & Bauer KA. (2005). Assessment of hemostatic risk factors in predicting arterial thrombotic events. *Arterioscler Thromb Vasc Biol,* Vol.25, No.10, pp.2043-53.

Fry, DL. (1968). Acute vascular endothelial changes associated with increased blood velocity gradients. *Circ Res.* Vol.22, No.2, pp.165-197.

Fuchs, TA., Brill, A., Duerschmied, D., Schatzberg, D., Monestier, M., Myers, DD, Jr, Wrobleski, SK., Wakefield, TW., Hartwig, JH., & Wagner, DD. (2010). Extracellular DNA traps promote thrombosis. *Proc Natl Acad Sci U S A.* Vol.107, No.36, pp.15880-15885.

Fukumoto, Y., Hiro, T., Fujii, T., Hashimoto, G., Fujimura, T., Yamada, J., Okamura, T., & Matsuzaki, M. (2008). Localized elevation of shear stress is related to coronary plaque rupture: a 3-dimensional intravascular ultrasound study with in-vivo color mapping of shear stress distribution. *J Am Coll Cardiol,* Vol.51, No.6, pp.645-650.

Gailani, D., & Broze, GJ Jr. (1991). Factor XI activation in a revised model of blood coagulation. *Science,* Vol.253, No.5022, pp.909-912.

Geiser, T., Sturzenegger, M., Genewein, U., Haeberli, A., & Beer, JH. (1998). Mechanisms of cerebrovascular events as assessed by procoagulant activity, cerebral microemboli, and platelet microparticles in patients with prosthetic heart valves. *Stroke,* Vol.29, No.9, pp.1770-1777.

Golino, P., Piscione, F., Willerson, JT., Cappelli-Bigazzi, M., Focaccio, A., Villari, B., Villari, B., Indolfi, C., Russolillo, E., Condorelli, M., & Chiariello, M. (1991). Divergent effects of serotonin on coronary-artery dimensions and blood flow in patients with coronary atherosclerosis and control patients. *N Engl J Med,* Vol.324, No.10, pp.641-648.

Hatakeyama, K., Asada, Y., Marutsuka, K., Sato, Y., Kamikubo, Y., & Sumiyoshi A. (1997). Localization and activity of tissue factor in human aortic atherosclerotic lesions. *Atherosclerosis,* Vol.133, No.2, pp.213-219.

Hill, JM., Zalos, G., Halcox, JP., Schenke, WH., Waclawiw, MA., Quyyumi, AA., & Finkel, T. (2003). Circulating endothelial progenitor cells, vascular function, and cardiovascular risk. *N Engl J Med,* Vol.348, No.7, pp.593-600.

Ishikawa, T., Hatakeyama, K., Imamura, T., Date, H., Shibata, Y., Hikichi, Y., Asada, Y., & Eto, T.(2003). Involvement of C-reactive protein obtained by directional coronary atherectomy in plaque instability and developing restenosis in patients with stable or unstable angina pectoris. *Am J Cardiol.* Vol.91, No.3, pp.287-292.

Kaikita, K., Soejima, K., Matsukawa, M., Nakagaki, T., & Ogawa, H. (2006). Reduced von Willebrand factor-cleaving protease (ADAMTS13) activity in acute myocardial infarction. *J Thromb Haemost.* Vol.4, No.11, pp.2490-2493.

Koike, T., Kitajima, S., Yu, Y., Nishijima, K., Zhang, J., Ozaki, Y., Morimoto, M., Watanabe, T., Bhakdi, S., Asada, Y., Chen, YE., & Fan, J. (2009). Human C-reactive protein does not promote atherosclerosis in transgenic rabbits. *Circulation,* Vol.120, No.21, pp.2088-2094.

Kolodgie, FD., Burke, AP., Farb, A., Gold, HK., Yuan, J., Narula, J., Finn, AV., & Virmani, R. (2001). The thin-cap fibroatheroma: a type of vulnerable plaque: the major precursor lesion to acute coronary syndromes. *Curr Opin Cardiol*, Vol.16, No.5, pp.285-292.

Kolodgie, FD., Gold, HK., Burke, AP., Fowler, DR., Kruth, HS., Weber, DK., Farb, A., Guerrero, LJ., Hayase, M., Kutys, R., Narula, J., Finn, AV., & Virmani, R. (2003). Intraplaque hemorrhage and progression of coronary atheroma. *N Engl J Med*, Vol.349, No.24, pp.2316-2325.

Kornecki, E., Ehrlich, YH., Egbring, R., Gramse, M., Seitz, R., Eckardt, A., Lukasiewicz, H., & Niewiarowski, S. (1988). Granulocyte-platelet interactions and platelet fibrinogen receptor exposure. *Am J Physiol*, Vol.255, No.3 Pt 2, pp.H651-658.

Kulkarni, S., Dopheide, SM., Yap, CL., Ravanat, C., Freund, M., Mangin, P., Heel, KA., Street, A., Harper, IS., Lanza, F., & Jackson, SP. (2000). A revised model of platelet aggregation. *J Clin Invest*. Vol.105, No.6, pp.783-791.

Lemkes, BA., Hermanides, J., Devries, JH., Holleman, F., Meijers, JC., & Hoekstra, JB. (2010). Hyperglycemia: a prothrombotic factor? *J Thromb Haemost*, Vol.8, No.8, pp.1663-1669.

Loree, HM., Kamm, RD., Atkinson, CM., & Lee, RT. (1991). Turbulent pressure fluctuations on surface of model vascular stenoses. *Am J Physiol*, Vol.261, No.3 Pt 2, pp.H644-H650.

Loree, HM., Kamm, RD., Stringfellow, RG., & Lee, RT. (1992). Effects of fibrous cap thickness on peak circumferential stress in model atherosclerotic vessels. Circ Res. Vol.71, No.4, pp.850-858.

Mackman, N. (2004). Role of tissue factor in hemostasis, thrombosis, and vascular development. *Arterioscler Thromb Vasc Biol*, Vol.24, No.6, pp.1015-1022.

Malek AM, Alper SL, & Izumo S. (1999). Hemodynamic shear stress and its role in atherosclerosis. *JAMA*. Vol.282, No.21, pp.2035-2042.

Marzilli, M., Sambuceti, G., Fedele, S., & L'Abbate A. (2000). Coronary microcirculatory vasoconstriction during ischemia in patients with unstable angina. *Am J Coll Cardiol*, Vol.35, No.2, pp.327-334.

Massberg, S., Konrad, I., Schürzinger, K., Lorenz, M., Schneider, S., Zohlnhoefer, D., Hoppe, K., Schiemann, M., Kennerknecht, E., Sauer, S., Schulz, C., Kerstan, S., Rudelius, M., Seidl, S., Sorge, F., Langer, H., Peluso, M., Goyal, P., Vestweber, D., Emambokus, NR., Busch, DH., Frampton, J., & Gawaz M. (2006). Platelets secrete stromal cell-derived factor 1alpha and recruit bone marrow-derived progenitor cells to arterial thrombi in vivo. *J Exp Med*, Vol.203, No.5, pp.1221-1233.

Massberg, S., Grahl, L., von Bruehl, ML., Manukyan, D., Pfeiler, S., Goosmann, C., Brinkmann, V., Lorenz, M., Bidzhekov, K., Khandagale, AB., Konrad, I., Kennerknecht, E., Reges, K., Holdenrieder, S., Braun, S., Reinhardt, C., Spannagl, M., Preissner, KT., & Engelmann, B. (2010). Reciprocal coupling of coagulation and innate immunity via neutrophil serine proteases. *Nat Med*, Vol.16, No.8, pp.887-896.

Matsuda, S., Yamashita, A., Sato, Y., Kitajima, S., Koike, T., Sugita, C., Moriguchi-Goto, S., Hatakeyama, K., Takahashi, M., Koshimoto, C., Matsuura, Y., Iwakiri, T., Chen, YE., Fan, J, & Asada Y. (2011). Human C-reactive protein enhances thrombus formation after neointimal balloon injury in transgenic rabbits. *J Thromb Haemost*, Vol.9, No.1, pp.201-208.

Miyamoto, S., Ogawa, H., Soejima, H., Takazoe, K., Kajiwara, I., Shimomura, H., Sakamoto, T., Yoshimura, M., Kugiyama, K., Yasue, H., & Ozaki Y. Enhanced platelet

aggregation in the coronary circulation after coronary spasm. *Thromb Res,* Vol.103, No.5, pp.377-386.
Moir, E., Robbie, LA., Bennett, B., & Booth, NA. (2002). Polymorphonuclear leucocytes have two opposing roles in fibrinolysis. *Thromb Haemost.* Vol.87, No.6, pp.1006-1010.
Moriguchi-Goto, S., Yamashita, A., Tamura, N., Soejima, K., Takahashi, M., Nakagaki, T., Goto, S., & Asada, Y. (2009). ADAMTS-13 attenuates thrombus formation on type I collagen surface and disrupted plaques under flow conditions. *Atherosclerosis,* Vol.203, No.2, pp.409-416.
Muller, JE., Tofler, GH., & Stone, PH. (1989). Circadian variation and triggers of onset of acute cardiovascular disease. *Circulation,* Vol.79, No.4, pp.733-743.
Nesbitt, WS., Westein, E., Tovar-Lopez, FJ., Tolouei, E., Mitchell, A., Fu, J., Carberry, J., Fouras, A., Jackson, & SP. (2009). A shear gradient-dependent platelet aggregation mechanism drives thrombus formation. *Nat Med.*Vol.15, No.,6 pp.665-673.
Nishihira, K., Yamashita, A., Tanaka, N., Kawamoto, R., Imamura, T., Yamamoto, R., Eto, T., & Asada, Y. (2006a). Inhibition of 5-hydroxytryptamine receptor prevents occlusive thrombus formation on neointima of the rabbit femoral artery. *J Thromb Haemost,* Vol.4, No.1, pp.247-255.
Nishihira, K., Imamura, T., Yamashita, A., Hatakeyama, K., Shibata, Y., Nagatomo, Y., Manabe, I., Nagai, R., Kitamura, K., & Asada, Y. (2006b). Increased expression of interleukin-10 in unstable plaque obtained by directional coronary atherectomy. *Eur Heart J.* Vol.27, No.2, pp.685-689.
Nishihira, K., Imamura, T., Hatakeyama, K., Yamashita, A., Shibata, Y., Date, H., Manabe, I., Nagai, R., Kitamura, K., & Asada, Y. (2007). Expression of interleukin-18 in coronary plaque obtained by atherectomy from stable and unstable angina. *Thromb Res,* Vol.121, No.2, pp.275-279.
Nishihira, K., Yamashita, A., Tanaka, N., Moriguchi-Goto, S., Imamura, T., Ishida, T., Kawashima, S., Yamamoto, R., Kitamura, K., & Asada, Y. (2008a). Serotonin induces vasoconstriction of smooth muscle cell-rich neointima through 5-hydroxytryptamine2A receptor in rabbit femoral arteries. *J Thromb Haemost,* Vol.6, No.7, pp.1207-1214.
Nishihira, K., Yamashita, A., Imamura, T., Hatakeyama, K., Sato, Y., Nakamura, H., Yodoi, J., Ogawa, H., Kitamura, K., & Asada, Y. (2008b). Thioredoxin in coronary culprit lesions: possible relationship to oxidative stress and intraplaque hemorrhage. *Atherosclerosis,* Vol.201, No.2, pp.360-367.
Nishihira, K., Yamashita, A., Ishikawa, T., Hatakeyama, K., Shibata, Y., & Asada Y. (2010). Composition of thrombi in late drug-eluting stent thrombosis versus de novo acute myocardial infarction. *Thromb Res,* Vol.126, No.3, pp.254-257.
Okada, K., Ueda, Y., Matsuo, K., Nishio, M., Hirata, A., Kashiwase, K., Asai, M., Nemoto, T., & Kodama, K. (2011). Frequency and healing of nonculprit coronary artery plaque disruptions in patients with acute myocardial infarction. *Am J Cardiol,* Vol.107, No.10, pp.1426-1429.
Oshima, S., Yasue, H., Ogawa, H., Okumura, K., & Matsuyama, K. (1990). Fibrinopeptide A is released into the coronary circulation after coronary spasm. *Circulation.* Vol.82, No.6, pp.2222-2225.
Owens, AP, 3rd, & Mackman, N. (2010). Tissue factor and thrombosis: The clot starts here. *Thromb Haemost,* Vol.104, No.3, pp.432-439.
Østerud, B. (2010). Tissue factor expression in blood cells. Thromb Res. Vol.125, Suppl 1, pp.S31-34.

Palabrica, T., Lobb, R., Furie, BC., Aronovitz, M., Benjamin, C., Hsu, YM., Sajer, SA., & Furie, B. (1992). Leukocyte accumulation promoting fibrin deposition is mediated in vivo by P-selectin on adherent platelets. *Nature,* Vol.359, No.6398, pp.848-851.

Rábai, G., Szilágyi, N., Sótonyi, P., Kovalszky, I., Szabó, L., Machovich, R., & Kolev, K. (2010). Contribution of neutrophil elastase to the lysis of obliterative thrombi in the context of their platelet and fibrin content. *Thromb Res,* Vol.126, No.2, pp.e94-101.

Reininger AJ, Bernlochner I, Penz SM, Ravanat C, Smethurst P, Farndale RW, Gachet C, Brandl R, & Siess W. (2010). A 2-step mechanism of arterial thrombus formation induced by human atherosclerotic plaques. *J Am Coll Cardiol.* 2010 Vol.55, No.11, pp.1147-1158.

Ridker, PM. (2007). C-reactive protein and the prediction of cardiovascular events among those at intermediate risk: moving an inflammatory hypothesis toward consensus. *J Am Coll Cardiol.* Vol.49, No.21, pp.2129-2138.

Rosito, GA., D'Agostino, RB., Massaro, J., Lipinska, I., Mittleman, MA., Sutherland, P., Wilson, PW., Levy, D., Muller, JE., & Tofler, GH. (2004). Association between obesity and a prothrombotic state: the Framingham Offspring Study. *Thromb Haemost,* Vol.91, No.4, pp.683-689.

Sato, Y., Hatakeyama, K., Yamashita, A., Marutsuka, K., Sumiyoshi, A., & Asada Y. (2005). Proportion of fibrin and platelets differs in thrombi on ruptured and eroded coronary atherosclerotic plaques in humans. *Heart,* Vol.91, No.4, pp.526-530.

Sato, Y., Hatakeyama, K., Marutsuka, K., & Asada Y. (2009). Incidence of asymptomatic coronary thrombosis and plaque disruption: comparison of non-cardiac and cardiac deaths among autopsy cases. *Thromb Res,* Vol.124, No.1, pp.19-23.

Schwartz, RS., Burke, A., Farb, A., Kaye, D., Lesser, JR., Henry, TD., & Virmani, R. (2009). Microemboli and microvascular obstruction in acute coronary thrombosis and sudden coronary death: relation to epicardial plaque histopathology. *J Am Coll Cardiol,* Vol.54, No.23, pp.2167-2173.

Shah, PK. (2003). Mechanisms of plaque vulnerability and rupture. *J Am Coll Cardiol,* Vol.41, No.4 Suppl S, pp.15S-22S.

Shida, Y., Nishio, K., Sugimoto, M., Mizuno, T., Hamada, M., Kato, S., Matsumoto, M., Okuchi, K., Fujimura, Y., & Yoshioka, A. (2008). Functional imaging of shear-dependent activity of ADAMTS13 in regulating mural thrombus growth under whole blood flow conditions. *Blood.* Vol.111, No.3, pp.1295-1298.

Singh, N., Gemmell, CH., Daly, PA., & Yeo, EL. (1995). Elevated platelet-derived microparticle levels during unstable angina. *Can J Cardiol,* Vol.11, No.11, pp.1015-1021.

Stary, HC., Chandler, AB., Dinsmore, RE., Fuster, V., Glagov, S., Insull, W. Jr., Rosenfeld, ME., Schwartz, CJ., Wagner, WD., & Wissler, RW. (1995). A definition of advanced types of atherosclerotic lesions and a histological classification of atherosclerosis. A report from the Committee on Vascular Lesions of the Council on Arteriosclerosis, American Heart Association. *Arterioscler Thromb Vasc Biol,* Vol.15, No.9, pp.1512-1531.

Sumi, T., Yamashita, A., Matsuda, S., Goto, S., Nishihira, K., Furukoji, E., Sugimura, H., Kawahara, H., Imamura, T., Kitamura, K., Tamura, S., & Asada, Y. (2010). Disturbed blood flow induces erosive injury to smooth muscle cell-rich neointima and promotes thrombus formation in rabbit femoral artery. *J Thromb Haemost.* Vol.8, No.6, pp.1394-1402.

Sun, H., Koike, T., Ichikawa, T., Hatakeyama, K., Shiomi, M., Zhang, B., Kitajima, S., Morimoto, M., Watanabe, T., Asada, Y., Chen, YE., & Fan, J. (2005). C-reactive protein in atherosclerotic lesions: its origin and pathophysiological significance. *Am J Pathol*, Vol.167, No.4, pp.1139-1148.

Topol, EJ., & Yadav, JS. (2003). Recognition of the importance of embolization in atherosclerotic vascular disease. *Circulation*. Vol.101, No.5, pp.570-580.

Vandendries, ER., Furie, BC., & Furie, B. (2004). Role of P-selectin and PSGL-1 in coagulation and thrombosis. *Thromb Haemost*. Vol.92, No.3, pp.459-466.

Virmani, R., Burke, AP., Kolodgie, FD., & Farb, A. (2003). Pathology of the thin-cap fibroatheroma: a type of vulnerable plaque. *J Interv Cardiol*. Vol.16.No.3, pp.267-272.

Virmani, R., Kolodgie, FD., Burke, AP., Farb, A., & Schwartz, SM. (2000). Lessons from sudden coronary death: a comprehensive morphological classification scheme for atherosclerotic lesions. *Arterioscler Thromb Vasc Biol*, Vol.20, No.5, pp.1262-1275.

Waldo, SW., Li, Y., Buono, C., Zhao, B., Billings, EM., Chang, J., & Kruth, HS. (2008). Heterogeneity of human macrophages in culture and in atherosclerotic plaques. *Am J Pathol*, Vol.172, No.4, pp.1112-1126.

Wang, L., Miller, C., Swarthout, RF., Rao, M., Mackman, N., & Taubman, MB. (2009). Vascular smooth muscle-derived tissue factor is critical for arterial thrombosis after ferric chloride-induced injury. *Blood*. Vol.113, No.3, pp.705-713.

Wilcox, JN., Smith, KM., Schwartz, SM., & Gordon D. (1989). Localization of tissue factor in the normal vessel wall and in the atherosclerotic plaque. *Proc Natl Acad Sci U S A*, Vol.86, No.8, pp.2839-2843.

Yamashita, A., Asada, Y., Sugimura, H., Yamamoto, H., Marutsuka, K., Hatakeyama, K., Tamura, S., Ikeda, Y., & Sumiyoshi, A. (2003). Contribution of von Willebrand factor to thrombus formation on neointima of rabbit stenotic iliac artery under high blood-flow velocity. *Arterioscler Thromb Vasc Biol*, Vol.23, No.6, pp.1105-1110.

Yamashita, A., Furukoji, E., Marutsuka, K., Hatakeyama, K., Yamamoto, H., Tamura, S., Ikeda, Y., Sumiyoshi, A., & Asada, Y. (2004). Increased vascular wall thrombogenicity combined with reduced blood flow promotes occlusive thrombus formation in rabbit femoral artery. *Arterioscler Thromb Vasc Biol*, Vol.24, No.12, pp.2420-2424.

Yamashita, A., Sumi, T., Goto, S., Hoshiba, Y., Nishihira, K., & Kawamoto R, et al. (2006a). Detection of von Willebrand factor and tissue factor in platelets-fibrin rich coronary thrombi in acute myocardial infarction. *Am J Cardiol*, Vol.97, No.1, pp.26-28.

Yamashita, A., Nishihira, K., Kitazawa, T., Yoshihashi, K., Soeda, T., Esaki, K., Imamura, T., Hattori, K., & Asada, Y. (2006b). Factor XI contributes to thrombus propagation on injured neointima of the rabbit iliac artery. *J Thromb Haemost*, Vol.4, No.7, pp.1496-1501.

Yamashita, A., Matsuda, S., Matsumoto, T., Moriguchi-Goto, S., Takahashi, M., Sugita, C., Sumi, T., Imamura, T., Shima, M., Kitamura, K., & Asada, Y. (2009). Thrombin generation by intimal tissue factor contributes to thrombus formation on macrophage-rich neointima but not normal intima of hyperlipidemic rabbits. *Atherosclerosis*. Vol.206, No.2, pp.418-426.

Zeng, B., Bruce, D., Kril, J., Ploplis, V., Freedman, B., & Brieger, D. (2002). Influence of plasminogen deficiency on the contribution of polymorphonuclear leucocytes to fibrin/ogenolysis: studies in plasminogen knock-out mice. *Thromb Haemost*. Vol.88, No.5, pp.805-810.

2

Biomarkers of Atherosclerosis and Acute Coronary Syndromes – A Clinical Perspective

Richard Body[1], Mark Slevin[2,3] and Garry McDowell[4,5]
[1]*Cardiovascular Sciences Research Group, University of Manchester, Manchester,*
[2]*School of Biology, Chemistry and Health Science, John Dalton Building, Manchester Metropolitan University, Manchester,*
[3]*Cardiovascular Research Centre, CSIC-ICCC, Hospital de la Santa Creu i Sant Pau, Barcelona,*
[4]*Faculty of Health, Edge Hill University, Ormskirk,*
[5]*School of Translational Medicine, University of Manchester, Manchester,*
[1,2,4,5]*UK*
[3]*Spain*

1. Introduction

Coronary heart disease remains the single biggest killer in the United Kingdom, accounting for around one in five deaths in men and one in six deaths in women (1). In 2003 the total annual cost of coronary heart disease in the United Kingdom was around £3.5 billion (£60 per capita), with the cost of inpatient care accounting for around 79% of these costs (2). Approximately 3% of patients who attend the ED have chest pain that the treating physician suspects may be cardiac in origin (3). 74-88% of these patients are admitted to hospital, making up one in five of all medical admissions (3-5). Ultimately only a quarter of these patients will be diagnosed with an acute coronary syndrome (ACS), which implies that a very cautious approach to the problem has been adopted. Despite this fact, up to 6% of the patients with chest pain who are discharged from the ED actually have myocardial damage that has prognostic significance (6). These patients are up to three times as likely to die as similar patients who were admitted to hospital (7).

2. The pathophysiology of coronary heart disease

Over the past century tremendous advances have been made in our understanding of coronary heart disease and its pathophysiological evolution. In 1910 a Russian physician first described the clinical presentation of acute myocardial infarction (AMI) (8). Two years later, an association was drawn between AMI and acute thrombotic coronary occlusion (9). By 1913 it had been hypothesised that atherosclerosis developed as a result of gradual lipid accumulation within the arterial wall (10). The advent of coronary revascularisation procedures in the latter half of the 20th century allowed the observation that restoring blood flow beyond significant coronary stenotic lesions often led to alleviation of anginal symptoms. This helped to propagate the widespread belief that the greater the coronary stenosis the greater the risk of a clinically significant event such as AMI or unstable angina pectoris. This axiom underpins much of modern practice in cardiology. Figure 1 illustrates the traditional model of the evolution of coronary atheroma (11).

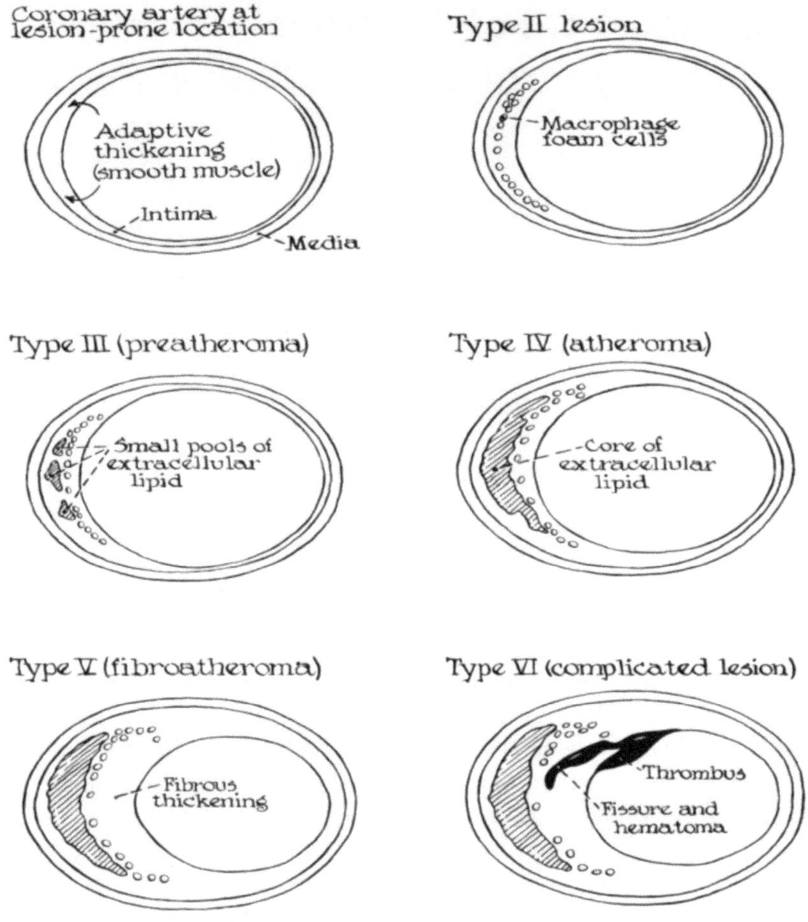

Fig. 1. Drawings of cross sections of the most proximal parts of six left anterior descending coronary arteries, illustrated to depict the traditional concept of the evolution of coronary atheroma. From Stary *et al*, 1995 (11).

In recent years this whole concept has been challenged. Far from a bland disease of cholesterol storage characterised by a passive accumulation of lipid within the vessel wall, a growing body of research and a progression in current thinking suggest that coronary atherosclerosis is in fact a dynamic inflammatory disease, dependent upon complex interactions between the immune, coagulation and humoral systems. It would seem that progression of coronary atherosclerosis is not so much a gradual process as a stepwise one, often characterised by swift and sudden increases in plaque size. Atherosclerotic plaque rupture or endothelial damage may lead to haemorrhage into the plaque or thrombus formation with subsequent organisation. This leads to rapid expansion of the plaque (12). Further, the severity of coronary stenosis on angiography does not predict the development of subsequent AMI (13). Indeed, two thirds of AMIs are provoked by plaques that cause less than 50% stenosis on angiography (14). The explanation for these phenomena resides in the understanding that there are, in basic terms, two kinds of coronary atheromatous plaques: those which are stable and those which are unstable. While stable plaques may be responsible for stable anginal symptoms (such as exertional chest pain relieved by rest), they are less likely to rupture and cause the clinical manifestations that we recognise as ACS. Meanwhile, unstable plaques are vulnerable and highly likely to rupture with the ensuing risk of developing ACS. There are notable pathological differences between these two types of plaque. Stable plaques are more likely to cause coronary stenosis, presenting a fixed obstruction to blood flow and therefore often being responsible for causing stable anginal symptoms such as exertional chest pain. Unstable plaques, however, may cause little arterial stenosis, thus explaining the observation that the majority of AMIs are caused by lesions that are only mildly stenotic. What is more, they may cause little in the way of clinical symptoms until they rupture, leading to the often dramatic and frequently fatal clinical manifestations of ACS.

Pathologically, stable plaques are likely to be more enriched with smooth muscle cells than those which are prone to rupture. They are likely to contain a dense fibrous cap consisting of collagen and extracellular matrix, which give the plaque tensile strength. On the contrary, plaques that are vulnerable to rupture are likely to have thin, friable fibrous caps, contain abundant inflammatory cells including macrophages and they are rich in extracellular lipid, often with a lipid core containing pro-inflammatory oxygen free radicals, pro-thrombotic material such as tissue factor and necrotic cellular debris (Figure 2) (15;16).

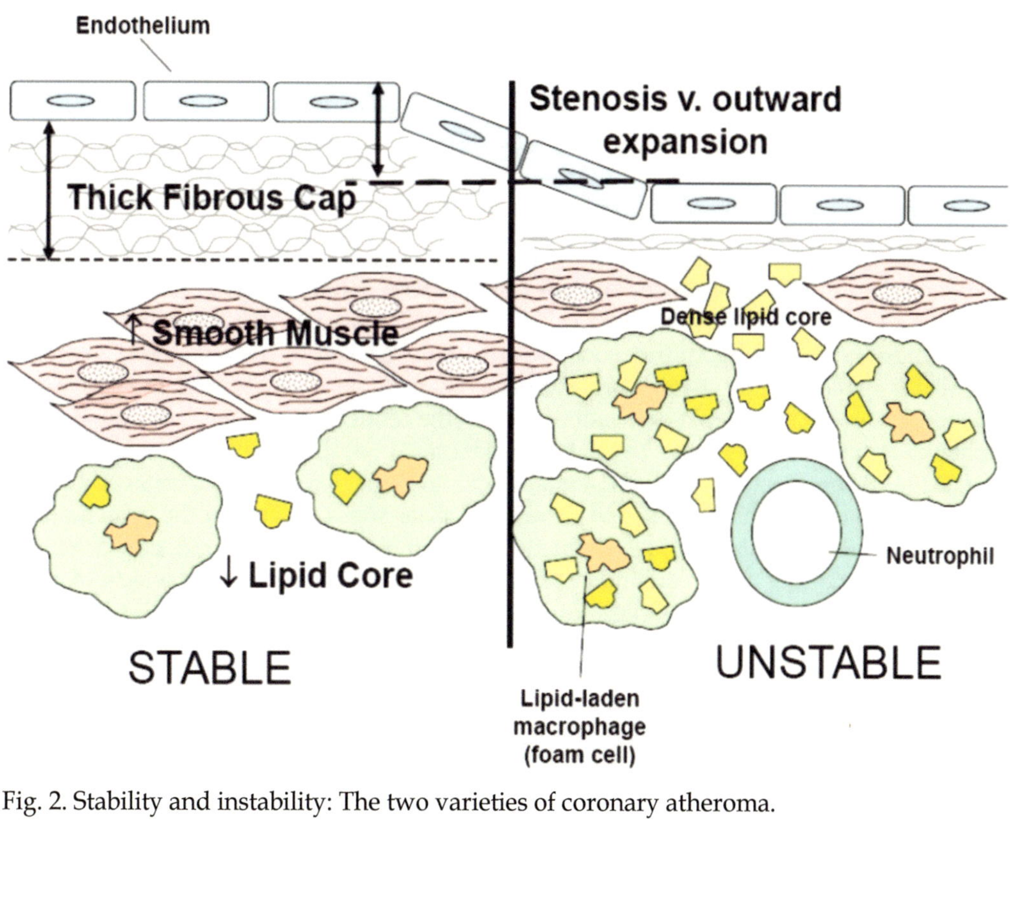

Fig. 2. Stability and instability: The two varieties of coronary atheroma.

While an unstable plaque often causes little or no arterial stenosis, it does not follow that unstable plaques are necessarily smaller in size than their stable counterparts. It has become apparent that the arterial wall is not a static and rigid structure but rather is capable of so-called 'outward remodelling', increasing its external diameter without narrowing the lumen. An unstable plaque may therefore be comparatively large in size while causing little arterial stenosis (15;17-21).

2.1 The pathophysiological evolution of an acute coronary syndrome

In order to fully comprehend the limitations to current diagnostic strategies and to attempt the development of effective new strategies for the diagnosis of ACS it is important to have a reasonable understanding of the initiation and progression of the disease from a molecular level upwards. If we can recognise the precise disease processes we are trying to accurately identify, we stand a much better chance of understanding our current problems and of developing effective novel diagnostic strategies that can be applied in clinical practice.

Coronary atherosclerosis is an inflammatory disease whose origins can only be adequately understood through a sound appreciation of vascular biology (17;22-27). We no longer regard the blood vessel wall as simply an inert tubular conduit for flowing blood but rather as a complex living structure that plays a pivotal role in maintaining vascular homeostasis and integrity. Of particular importance in this regard is the endothelium, a monolayer of cells forming a barrier between flowing blood and tissue. The human endothelium has a total surface area of approximately $1000m^2$ (16) and constitutes around 16% of the myocardium (28). It plays a key role in modulating vascular tone, responding to neural, humoral and mechanical stimuli by synthesising and releasing vasoactive substances. By sending activating signals to circulating inflammatory cells, the endothelium orchestrates complex fluid and cellular movements designed to neutralise and eliminate foreign elements. While these mechanisms are usually beneficial, under certain circumstances these processes can become extreme and counter-productive (29;30).

The endothelium is an active player in the protection against and development of coronary disease, being the guardian of the integrity of the vessel wall. A functional endothelium produces a healthy balance of vascular constricting and relaxing factors. In this respect, the role of endothelium-derived nitric oxide is particularly crucial. In addition to its important vasodilator effect, nitric oxide protects against vascular injury, inflammation and thrombosis. It inhibits leukocyte adhesion to the endothelium, smooth muscle cell proliferation and migration and platelet aggregation (31-34). In the presence of traditional cardiac risk factors such as hyperlipidaemia, smoking, diabetes and hypertension and where there is local or systemic inflammation or reduced shear stress (such as at the branch points of coronary arteries), nitric oxide production is inhibited and its degradation enhanced (Figure 3) (23). Under these conditions, many of the protective inhibitory effects of nitric oxide are lost. Cell adhesion molecules (CAMs) including P-selectin and E-selectin are expressed by the endothelium, where they mediate leukocyte binding. P-selectin and E-selectin bind to carbohydrates that are constitutively expressed on the surface of circulating leukocytes, causing the leukocytes to bind loosely to the endothelial surface and to literally roll across it, scanning the endothelium for further activating signals. Chemoattractant cytokines or chemokines that are also expressed by activated endothelial cells can then induce a conformational change in integrin molecules expressed at the leukocyte cell surface, changing them from a low-affinity to a high-affinity state (35). These activated integrins may then bind firmly to two further adhesion molecules that are expressed by activated endothelium: intercellular adhesion molecule-1 (ICAM-1) and vascular cellular adhesion molecule-1 (VCAM-1). This strong adhesion brings the rolling leukocytes to a halt.

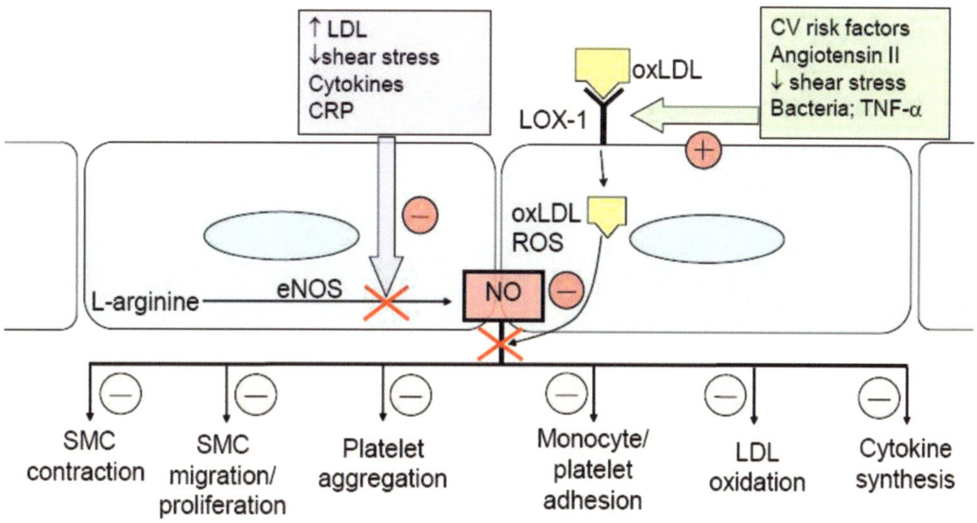

Fig. 3. The pivotal anti-atherogenic role of nitric oxide on a molecular level. Abbreviations: LDL, low density lipoprotein; CRP, C-reactive protein; CV, cardiovascular; TNF- α, tumour necrosis factor α; oxLDL, oxidised LDL; ROS, reactive oxygen species; SMC, smooth muscle cell; NO, nitric oxide; LOX-1, oxidised LDL receptor-1; eNOS, endothelial nitric oxide synthase.

In the presence of further activating signals from within the arterial intima, the leukocytes may subsequently undergo a cytoskeletal change, enabling them to squeeze between the tight cell-cell junctions of the endothelium via interactions with the PECAM-1 (CD31) receptor. Again, under normal circumstances PECAM-1 binds endothelial cells strongly together, preventing leukocyte migration into the arterial intima. However, substances such as thrombin and histamine that are expressed during periods of localised inflammation loosen this binding, promoting cellular retraction and vascular permeability. This enables glycoproteins on the cell surface of the activated leukocytes to bind to PECAM-1, allowing them to pass through the endothelial layer into the arterial intima in a process labelled diapedesis (29;36). Within the arterial intima, activated leukocytes will then migrate towards chemokines (including monocyte chemotactic protein, MCP-1) expressed within foci of inflammation where they participate in inflammatory processes (Figure 4) (29;37;38).

Circulating low-density lipoprotein (LDL) cholesterol can also bind to endothelial receptors and is subsequently modified or oxidised by the endothelial cells. Within the arterial intima, oxidised LDL acts as a strong stimulus for further migration and localisation of inflammatory cells (16). Following migration, monocytes mature into macrophages and, via scavenger receptors, ingest oxidised LDL to become foam cells (24). Together with T lymphocytes and activated endothelial cells, these cells secrete an array of pro-inflammatory cytokines, forming a positive feedback loop which enhances the inflammatory reaction within the arterial intima. If the inflammatory stimuli are not removed or neutralised, this process will continue indefinitely (27).

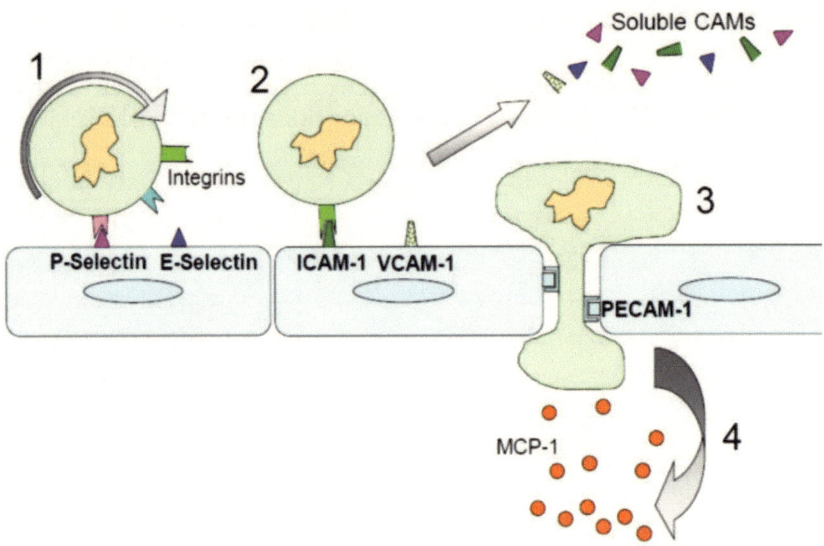

Fig. 4. The multistep model of leukocyte migration. 1. Leukocytes bind to selectins expressed by activated endothelium, causing them to roll, scanning the endothelium for activating signals. 2. In the presence of activating signals, integrins on the cell surface of the leukocyte undergo a structural change and can bind firmly to ICAM-1 and VCAM-1. 3. Leukocytes can then migrate through to the arterial intima by binding to PECAM-1 at the cell junction. 4. Leukocytes migrate along a chemokine gradient (illustrated as MCP-1), which helps to localise the inflammatory response within the intima. Cell adhesion molecules are subsequently released into the circulation in soluble form.

In addition to enhancing inflammation, cytokines stimulate differentiation and migration of smooth muscle cells from the arterial media into the intima (39). While this may ultimately lead to mechanical expansion of the plaque, smooth muscle cells actually play a vital role in maintaining the stability of the atherosclerotic plaque by secreting a dense, fibrous extracellular matrix and substances that prevent its degradation (tissue inhibitors of metalloproteinases, TIMPs) (16) (Figure 5).

Enhanced inflammatory activity within the plaque ultimately renders the plaque vulnerable to rupture by destabilising this fibrous cap. Activated macrophages and neutrophils within atheroma secrete myeloperoxidase (MPO), an enzyme which enhances consumption of nitric oxide, generating highly reactive and pro-inflammatory oxygen free radicals and oxidised LDL, thus perpetuating and enhancing both endothelial dysfunction and the formation of foam cells (40;41). MPO inactivates TIMPs, paving the way for degradation of the fibrous cap. Further, MPO activates matrix metalloproteinases (MMPs), enzymes responsible for actively degrading the fibrous cap (42) (Figure 6) (43).

Atheroma is rendered even more vulnerable to rupture by interactions between the CD40 receptor (which is expressed by endothelial cells, monocytes and B lymphocytes) and its ligand CD40L, which is expressed by activated T helper cells, smooth muscle cells, macrophages, basophils and activated platelets (44;45). This interaction leads to the formation of another positive feedback loop that enhances endothelial dysfunction and inflammation within the plaque and stimulates the release of both the procoagulant tissue factor and MMPs into the lipid core (46-50). The latter further enhance degradation of the fibrous cap (Figure 6).

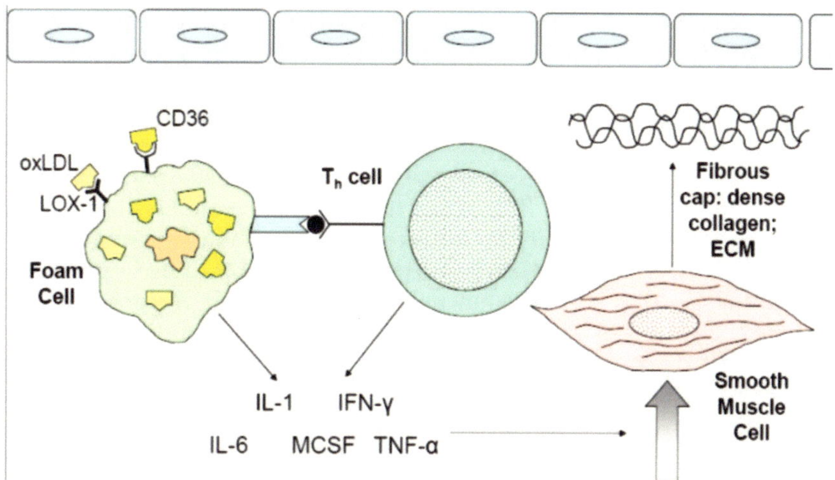

Fig. 5. Progression to organised atheroma. Following migration into the arterial intima, monocytes mature into tissue macrophages and, via receptors including LOX-1 and CD36, take up extracellular lipid including oxidised LDL cholesterol (oxLDL) to become foam cells. Together with T helper cells (Th), foam cells secrete an array of pro-inflammatory cytokines (interleukin-1 (IL-1), interferon-γ (IFN-γ), interleukin-6 (IL-6), monocyte colony stimulating factor (MCSF), tumour necrosis factor- α (TNF- α)), which lead to migration of vascular smooth muscle cells from the arterial media. Following migration, these smooth muscle cells secrete a dense extracellular matrix (ECM) and collagen fibres, which form a tough fibrous cap.

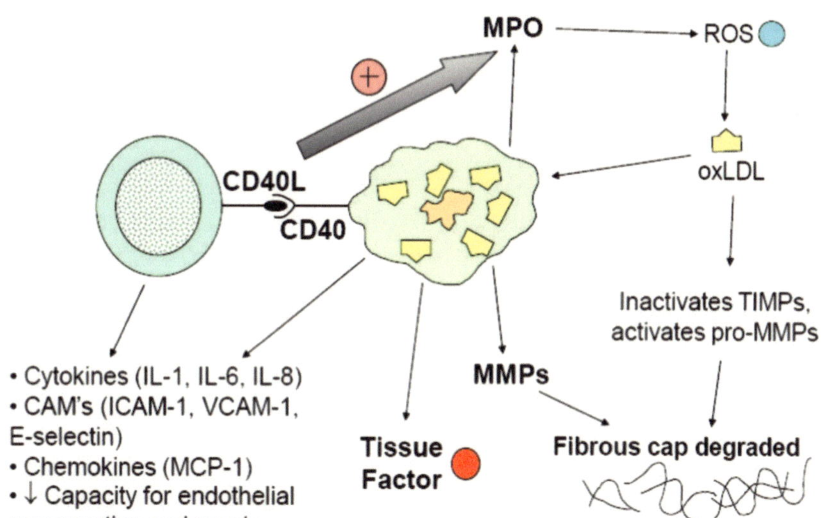

Fig. 6. CD40/L interactions within coronary atheroma. CD40/40L interactions lead to enhanced inflammation, impaired capacity for endothelial repair and regeneration, secretion of pro-coagulant tissue factor, MMPs and upregulation of myeloperoxidase (MPO) secretion. MPO produces reactive oxygen species (ROS) and oxidised LDL (oxLDL), enhancing upregulation and leading to degradation of the fibrous cap by activating the precursors of MMPs (pro-MMPS) and inhibiting tissue inhibitors of metalloproteinases (TIMPs).

Where there is abundant intimal inflammation, pro-inflammatory cytokines may prime cells within the plaque for apoptotic death upon engagement with activated T lymphocytes (22;51). Stimulated apoptosis of smooth muscle cells impedes maintenance of the fibrous cap, favouring its breakdown. Apoptosis of endothelial cells may lead to erosions of the endothelial layer, enabling circulating blood to come into contact with the pro-thrombotic contents of the plaque (Figure 7). Circulating platelets are activated upon contact, binding to the arterial wall and to each other (52). When these areas of endothelial erosion are small, this platelet aggregation occurs only on a microscopic level and is clinically insignificant, serving only to stimulate endothelial regeneration and smooth muscle growth. The new endothelial cells may be dysfunctional, however, predisposing to vasoconstriction (15).

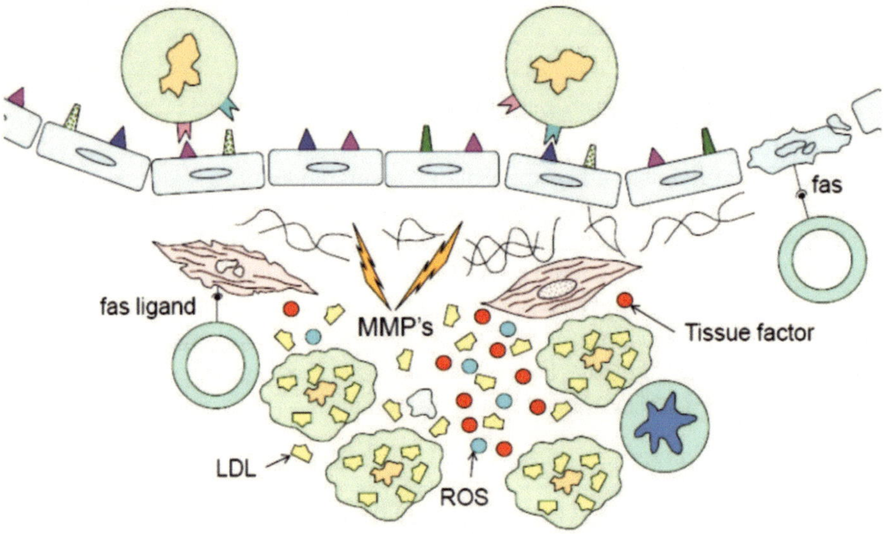

Fig. 7. Positive feedback loops within unstable coronary atheroma and processes leading to endothelial erosion.

In the presence of larger endothelial erosions there may be a rapid increase in intimal inflammation (53) and sufficient platelet aggregation and subsequent fibrin deposition to produce a large thrombus with symptomatic luminal obstruction (15;17;54;55). In itself, this process accounts for approximately 25% of all major thrombi that lead to acute coronary syndromes (56) and may have even greater importance in women and young people (57). Of even greater importance, however, is the high tensile stress that a vulnerable plaque must withstand. As the lipid core is soft and deformable, it cannot bear circumferential stress. This stress is therefore borne by the fibrous cap, made of tough collagen and extracellular matrix. Depending upon the shape of the plaque and its position within the artery, the fibrous cap must withstand focal concentrations of load up to seven or eight times normal systolic wall stress (58;59). This is particularly significant in unstable plaques where the fibrous cap may be thin and friable.

Ultimately, this may lead to sudden rupture of the plaque with endothelial disruption, causing haemorrhage of circulating blood into the core of the plaque (Figure 8). This may be particularly likely to occur following a trigger such as unaccustomed physical activity or emotional stress, which leads to a rapid increase in systolic blood pressure and thus increased circumferential stress on an already vulnerable plaque (60).

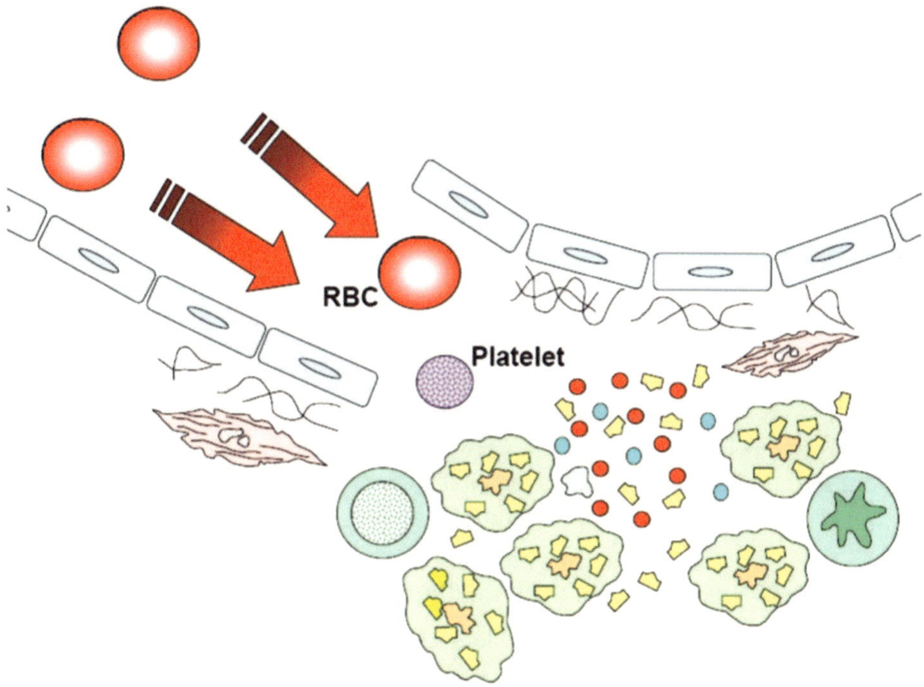

Fig. 8. Plaque rupture. There is haemorrhage into the plaque, causing rapid expansion and, as the contents of the lipid core are highly prothrombotic, thrombus formation ensues. Abbreviations: RBC, red blood cell.

Circulating blood is exposed to the prothrombotic lipid core. Tissue factor activates factor VIIa, which ultimately leads to the cleavage of thrombin from prothrombin and further activation of the coagulation cascade (61). Several substances from within the plaque, including thrombin, CD40L and P-selectin, activate circulating platelets by inducing a conformational change in the glycoprotein receptors and enabling cross-linking or adhesion via fibrinogen and other adhesive ligands. During this process, activated platelets themselves express P-selectin and CD40L, which appear to be necessary for the formation of a stable arterial thrombus (62-64). Both P-selectin and CD40L are later enzymatically cleaved from the platelet surface and released into the circulation in soluble form (65;66).

When plaque rupture is small, intraplaque haemorrhage may lead to rapid expansion with platelet activation and adhesion but the thrombus does not extend into the arterial lumen (12). The thrombus subsequently undergoes organisation, the endothelial layer regenerates and the episode is clinically silent. Among patients with coronary atheroma who died of non-vascular causes such as motor vehicle accidents and subsequently underwent post-mortem examination, up to 8% were noted to have had a recent plaque disruption with intra-plaque thrombi (67). Indeed, in pathological studies of subjects who died of ischaemic heart disease each patient had on average two to three plaque disruptions, although in each case one culprit thrombus was identified that was apparently responsible for causing death (68-70). In the presence of a large plaque rupture or, indeed, when the rupture is not large but the patient is in a pro-thrombotic state (for example during periods of stress or systemic infection), platelet activation and aggregation may extend into the arterial lumen. Activation of the coagulation cascade leads to fibrin deposition, which increases the size of the thrombus. Again, thrombus formation may be arrested without causing significant luminal stenosis. However, as the thrombus is exposed to flowing blood distal emboli may occur, potentially causing myocardial necrosis on a microscopic level and recognisable symptoms. As activated platelets aggregate to form a platelet-rich arterial thrombus, they release mediators such as serotonin and thromboxane A2, which cause vasoconstriction. This may lead to localised coronary arterial spasm, which even in the absence of an obstructive coronary thrombus, may lead to transmural myocardial ischaemia and a clinically apparent ACS (71). When thrombus formation continues unchecked, total arterial occlusion may occur. If such occlusion occurs suddenly in a previously uncompromised artery without a well-developed collateral circulation, significant downstream myocardial necrosis will occur with the clinically recognisable signs of acute myocardial infarction (AMI). The cell membranes of the necrosed myocytes are breached and their intracellular constituents are washed out into the circulation. These constituents include myoglobin, creatine kinase, the cardiac troponins and human fatty acid binding protein.

3. Biomarkers of unstable coronary disease

Current diagnostic strategies incorporate biomarkers of myocardial necrosis, the end-point in the pathophysiological evolution of ACS. The measurement of cardiac troponins in the bloodstream has revolutionised the diagnosis of AMI in this regard, enabling the detection of microscopic amounts of myocardial necrosis that could not have previously been identified (72). As described in detail earlier in this chapter, however, a whole host of pathophysiological processes have occurred before myocardial necrosis, none of which are detectable using current diagnostic technology. In fact myocardial necrosis is merely a surrogate marker of the disease process, which occurs within the coronary artery and not the cardiac myocyte. As it is possible to use biomarkers to detect myocardial necrosis with high sensitivity and specificity this raises the additional possibility that other biomarkers may be able to detect evidence of the disease process itself within the coronary arteries. A number of novel biomarkers have been investigated in this regard in recent years.

3.1 Soluble cell adhesion molecules

Cell adhesion molecules (CAMs) mediate the interactions between the endothelium and blood cells, enabling the localised inflammatory response that is essential for the initiation and propagation of coronary atherosclerosis. Their upregulation enhances this inflammatory response, which ultimately renders the atherosclerotic plaque vulnerable to rupture. Following their expression, CAMs are shed from the cell surface. As these soluble CAMs are detectable in peripheral blood, they are promising candidates for use as early markers of vascular activation (37). CAMs that have attracted interest as potential biomarkers of ACS include the molecules P-selectin, E-selectin, ICAM-1 and VCAM-1.

3.1.1 P-selectin

P-selectin mediates the interaction of platelets and endothelial cells with neutrophils and monocytes (65). It is expressed by endothelial cells in atherosclerotic, but not normal, vessels

(73,74), with expression being particularly marked in patients with unstable angina (75). P-selectin is also expressed by activated platelets and has been used as a marker of platelet activation (76). Several investigators have demonstrated significantly raised soluble P-selectin levels in patients with AMI (77-84), unstable angina (85-88) and cohorts of patients with any ACS (89,90). However conflicting results have also been reported, with two reports that P-selectin does not help to predict adverse events in patients with ACS and two studies that did not detect any elevation of plasma P-selectin levels in patients with ACS compared with controls (91-93).

Five studies have investigated the utility of P-selectin for diagnosis of ACS in the ED population. One small study of 44 patients found no different in plasma soluble P-selectin levels between patients diagnosed with ACS and non-cardiac pain (94). Although the same group also reported that P-selectin was not an independent predictor for a diagnosis of ACS (95), another group reported that P-selectin was an independent predictor for the occurrence of serious cardiac events within three months of presentation to the ED with chest pain (96). Other groups have reported sensitivities of 35 and 55.8% and NPVs of 53 and 71% for the diagnosis of ACS (97-98). The data suggests that the use of soluble P-selectin as a sole rule-out strategy for ACS in the ED is likely to lead to an unacceptably high false negative rate. Our own data however in 713 patients presenting to the ED with suspected cardiac chest pain demonstrated P-selectin had early diagnostic value for AMI and prognostic significance independent of troponin T and ECG findings (99)

3.1.2 E-selectin

E-selectin has also been investigated in this regard. Plasma levels of E-selectin have been shown to correlate with the severity of coronary atherosclerosis (87,100). A number of studies have reported elevated plasma E-selectin levels in patients with AMI (101-108). E-selectin elevations have also been reported in patients with unstable angina (85,109). Other studies have reported raised E-selectin in all ACS (80,82,110-112). Plasma E-selectin levels in patients with AMI may be higher among patients who experienced a prodrome of unstable angina (105). Raised E-selectin levels have also been reported following attacks of variant angina (113), although there may be no difference in E-selectin levels during episodes of stable angina (114). A reduction in plasma E-selectin levels has been described in patients with AMI following successful reperfusion (101,108). Further, plasma E-selectin levels may be useful for predicting the risk of death among patients with AMI (103). However not all reports have been consistent. Three groups have failed to find elevated E-selectin levels in ACS (115-117). There is no clear explanation for the discrepancy in the results, although one group measured E-selectin in serum rather than plasma, which may have introduced an important bias. Only one study has investigated E-selectin levels in the ED population with undifferentiated chest pain (118). This study failed to demonstrate a difference in E-selectin levels between patients with AMI, unstable angina and controls. However, the study had significant limitations, including small numbers, suboptimal gold standards and no clinical follow-up. The study was not designed to appraise the performance of E-selectin as a diagnostic test for use in the ED. The available research suggests that E-selectin has promising characteristics for use as a marker of ACS. A large prospective observational cohort study is necessary to evaluate its performance as a diagnostic test. Incorporation into a multimarker strategy with markers that may reflect other aspects of the pathophysiological evolution of ACS may be necessary to obtain sufficient sensitivity.

3.1.3 Intercellular Adhesion Molecule-1 (ICAM-1) and Vascular Cell Adhesion Molecule-1 (VCAM-1)

ICAM-1 and VCAM-1 are responsible for mediating firm adhesion of leukocytes to the endothelium, enabling their subsequent migration. ICAM-1 (but not VCAM-1) levels have been shown to predict adverse cardiac events in apparently healthy men (119-121) and women (122) and may help to predict the development (121,123) and progression of coronary atherosclerosis (124). In addition, ICAM-1 (but not VCAM-1) levels are raised in patients with stable angina and levels may correlate with disease severity (125-127). Levels of both VCAM-1 and ICAM-1 have been shown to be elevated in patients with ACS (128-129), although conflicting results have also been reported (130). Interestingly, levels of VCAM-1 and ICAM-1 in patients with unstable angina who had demonstrable ruptured plaque on coronary intravascular ultrasound were significantly higher than in patients with stable angina who had no evidence of plaque rupture, although neither biomarker was an independent predictor of plaque rupture on multivariate analysis (131). Finally, VCAM-1 and ICAM-1 levels have both been shown to predict prognosis and complications in patients with confirmed ACS (91,103,128,132-137). Evidence for the use of ICAM-1 and VCAM-1 in the ED population with undifferentiated chest pain is disappointing, however. A study of 241 men who presented to the ED with chest pain failed to find a significant difference in ICAM-1 and VCAM-1 levels between patients with AMI and patients with (presumed) non-cardiac chest pain, although the gold standards for diagnosis of non-cardiac pain were suboptimal (138). Other studies have demonstrated no correlation between ICAM-1 and VCAM-1 levels and the occurrence of adverse events within three months of presentation (96,139). One study demonstrated that ICAM-1 predicted in-hospital adverse events with a sensitivity of 63.3%, a specificity of 47.2% and a NPV of 79.3%, which is clearly not sufficient for ICAM-1 to be used in the clinical environment (140).

3.1.4 Soluble CD40 Ligand (sCD40L)

As described earlier in this chapter sCD40L plays a pivotal role in mediating interactions between inflammatory cells within coronary atheroma that ultimately render the plaque vulnerable to rupture. In addition, sCD40L is expressed by activated platelets and plasma levels have been shown to correlate with platelet activation (141). Case control studies have consistently demonstrated elevated levels of sCD40L in patients with ACS when compared with controls (48;141-151). sCD40L levels have also been shown to stratify patients with confirmed ACS according to their risk of developing adverse events (152), although conflicting results have also been reported (153,154). An analysis of data from 1088 patients with confirmed ACS who had been enrolled in a randomised controlled trial (the c7E3 Fab antiplatelet therapy in unstable refractory angina (CAPTURE) trial) and 626 patients who were admitted to hospital with acute chest pain, found that sCD40L was a powerful independent predictor of adverse events at 72 hours, 30 days and six months. Levels correlated poorly with troponin T and may thus identify a separate at-risk group. However sCD40L may be more useful for prognostication than diagnosis. Using the 97.5th percentile upper reference limit as a diagnostic cut-off sCD40L had a sensitivity of only 56.5% for the diagnosis of ACS in the patients with acute chest pain (141).

3.2 Myeloperoxidase (MPO)

MPO is an enzyme secreted by phagocytic cells. It utilises hydrogen peroxidise to generate oxygen free radicals. In health this leads to the generation of hypochlorous acid, which has bactericidal and viricidal properties (155). Neutrophils and foam cells within coronary atheroma also produce MPO, where the generation of highly reactive oxygen free radicals leads to the generation of oxidised LDL cholesterol, which enhances the formation of foam cells propagating inflammation (156). It also perpetuates the endothelial dysfunction by enhancing the breakdown of nitric oxide (155). Further, MPO activates MMPs from their precursors and inactivates their physiological inhibitors, TIMPS (42). This enables breakdown of the fibrous cap, rendering the plaque vulnerable to rupture. MPO is abundantly expressed by macrophages in eroded or ruptured coronary plaques, although it has not been identified in fatty streaks (43). While expression is enhanced in unstable angina and AMI, it is not enhanced in variant angina or in response to ischaemia in chronic stable angina (157). These findings suggest that increased MPO expression is associated with the ongoing inflammatory process rather than indicating reperfusion injury or a tissue response to ischaemia. Blood levels of MPO have been shown to correlate strongly with the presence of coronary artery disease. When divided into quartiles, patients with MPO levels in the fourth quartile had an adjusted odds ratio for the presence of coronary artery disease of 20.4 compared to patients in the first quartile. MPO levels were more predictive of risk of coronary artery disease than Framingham risk score (158).

A case control study involving 874 patients demonstrated elevated MPO levels in patients with ACS compared with controls who had normal coronary angiograms (159). Two separate analyses of data from randomised controlled trials, involving a total of 2,614 patients, have reported that MPO levels help to predict the occurrence of adverse events in patients with confirmed ACS. Interestingly MPO was found to add additional prognostic information to cardiac troponins. However the rate of major adverse events within 30 days in patients with MPO levels below selected cut-offs remained around 5% in both studies (160,161). Other studies have also demonstrated that MPO levels in patients with confirmed ACS help to predict prognosis (162-165) , although one study reported that MPO levels did not help to predict mortality among 325 male patients who had been admitted to hospital with chest pain and were awaiting coronary angiography (166). Several studies have investigated the use of MPO in the ED population. The largest study, of 604 consecutive patients presenting to the ED with suspected cardiac chest pain, found that MPO levels predicted a diagnosis of ACS with sensitivity 65.7%, specificity 60.7%, PPV 53.3%, and NPV 72.2%. MPO levels also predicted adverse events, although 14.8% of patients with normal MPO and troponin levels still had a major adverse event within 30 days (167). A second study of 414 low risk patients who presented to the ED with suspected ACS found that MPO had a sensitivity of 71%, specificity 32% and negative likelihood ratio 0.89 (95% CI 0.26 - 2.05), suggesting that MPO was not a useful diagnostic test for AMI. However the study was underpowered as only seven patients were diagnosed with ACS (168). Among 140 consecutive ED patients with chest pain, MPO helped to diagnose AMI with sensitivity 92.3% (CI 95% 66.7% - 99.6%), specificity 40.2% (CI 95% 32.0% - 48.9%), PPV 13.6% (CI 95%

8.0% - 22.3%) and NPV 98.1% (CI 95% 89.9% - 99.9%). Again, however, the study was underpowered, with only 13 patients being diagnosed with AMI (169). Finally, MPO levels measured in 148 ED patients with chest pain were found to be significantly higher among those diagnosed with AMI. However MPO was both insensitive (13.9% of patients with MPO levels in the bottom quartile had AMI) and non-specific as a diagnostic marker for AMI (only 38.4% of patients with values in the highest quartile had AMI). MPO levels were found to be significant predictors of adverse events within 30 days (167) The available data suggest that MPO is unlikely to have sufficient sensitivity or specificity to be useful as an early diagnostic marker of ACS in the ED. However it may have a role for risk stratification and prediction of prognosis, particularly in troponin negative patients.

3.3 Pregnancy-Associated Plasma Protein A (PAPP-A)

PAPP-A is a matrix metalloproteinase (MMP), one of a family of at least 25 proteases, of which 14 have been characterised in vascular cells. They are secreted by a variety of cells that are involved in the atherosclerotic process including foam cells, endothelial cells, T lymphocytes, mast cells and smooth muscle cells (170). They are upregulated in atherosclerotic plaque and play a pivotal role in the degradation of the fibrous cap that renders the plaque vulnerable to rupture (171,172). PAPP-A was originally detected in the serum in late pregnancy and has been used in first trimester screening for Down's syndrome (173). It is also abundantly expressed in unstable but not stable atherosclerotic plaques (54) and raised levels have been shown to correlate with complex coronary stenoses on angiography (174). A small case control study involving a total of 69 patients found that PAPP-A levels were significantly higher in patients with AMI or unstable angina compared to patients with stable angina and healthy controls without coronary disease (54). PAPP-A has been investigated as a potential early marker of AMI, with mixed results. A study of 346 patients who presented to the ED with chest pain found that PAPP-A levels were significantly higher in those patients who were diagnosed with AMI (175). In a second study that included 415 patients admitted to a cardiology unit with suspected ACS, PAPP-A levels were also found to be significantly higher in those patients with AMI although the AUC was only 0.56, suggesting that PAPP-A is unlikely to be useful as a lone diagnostic investigation for AMI (176). Further, a case control study found no significant difference in PAPP-A levels between 80 patients with STEMI and 80 healthy controls (177). Finally, among 59 patients who presented to the ED with suspected ACS and were deemed to be at intermediate risk for having a significant coronary event, PAPP-A was found to be an independent predictor of a diagnosis of ACS (odds ratio 2.09), following adjustment for other clinical factors (178).

When tested at the time of presentation in the ED population, PAPP-A may help to predict cardiac events in the near future. In a subgroup of a large study involving 626 ED patients with chest pain, Heeschen et al found that PAPP-A predicted adverse events with an adjusted odds ratio of 2.32 (179). In an ED population of 136 patients with suspected ACS but negative troponin I, Lund et al found PAPP-A to be an independent predictor of adverse cardiac events at six months, albeit with a sensitivity of only 54%, specificity 75%, PPV 30% and NPV 15% (180). In a study of 364 ED patients with suspected ACS, Laterza et al reported that PAPP-A predicted adverse events at 30 days with a sensitivity of 66.7%, specificity 51.5%, PPV 12.6% and NPV 93.6%. Thus for every 100 patients discharged and reassured on the basis of a negative PAPP-A level, three would have an adverse cardiac events within 30 days (175). Finally, among 422 patients who presented to the ED with chest pain but had neither troponin elevations nor ECG abnormalities, PAPP-A was found to be a significant predictor of adverse events after a median of 60 weeks follow up, although this was not significant once other factors had been taken into account (including a clinical risk score, exercise tolerance testing and plasma levels of other biomarkers) (181). The available evidence suggests that PAPP-A levels alone are unlikely to be sufficient to enable early diagnosis of AMI in the ED or to accurately identify a population of patients who are at sufficiently low risk of adverse events to affect clinical practice.

3.4 Coagulation markers

3.4.1 D-dimer

D-dimer is a degradation product of cross-linked fibrin. Its presence indicates both thrombus formation and subsequent endogenous fibrinolysis, thus confirming that both thrombin and plasmin have been generated (182). It is a sensitive tool for exclusion of venous thromboembolism in the low risk group (183). In ACS plaque rupture or erosion is followed by exposure of the procoagulant lipid core to circulating blood with ensuing thrombus formation. As coronary thrombus precedes myocardial necrosis, it is possible that coagulation markers such as D-dimer are sensitive markers of ACS, potentially rising earlier than markers of myocardial necrosis including troponins. Elevated D-dimer levels in apparently healthy males have been shown to predict the future occurrence of AMI, ACS and coronary heart disease (121,184,185). Further, patients in whom the first presentation of coronary heart disease is with AMI may have higher D-dimer levels than patients who first present with stable angina (186). A weak but statistically significant correlation has been demonstrated between plasma D-dimer levels and severity of coronary disease on angiography in patients with unstable angina (187,188). In a cohort of 54 patients who were diagnosed with unstable angina and underwent coronary angiography, D-dimer levels (cut-off 270ng/ml) predicted significant coronary disease on angiography with sensitivity 70%, specificity 50%, PPV 86%, NPV 72%. By lowering the cut-off to 200ng/ml sensitivity increased to 95% but specificity dropped to 20% (189).

Several studies have demonstrated that patients with ACS have elevated levels of D-dimer when compared to controls with stable angina or no coronary disease (139,190,193). Plasma D-dimer level has also been shown to be a significant predictor of long-term mortality (after a median of 29 months follow up) in 320 patients with a diagnosis of NSTE-ACS (194), although a separate study of 358 patients with NSTE-ACS found that D-dimer did not predict the occurrence of adverse events (death, AMI, revascularisation or hospital admission for acute heart failure) within six months (hazard ratio 1.26, 95% CI 0.79 - 2.02) (195). Among 257 patients D-dimer levels (cut-off 500ng/l) at the time of admission (mean 160 minutes from symptom onset) diagnosed AMI with sensitivity 65%, specificity 80%, PPV 36% and NPV 93%, although the study utilised an outdated gold standard (incorporating CK-MB levels) for the diagnosis of AMI. D-dimer levels were found to be significantly higher in patients who were diagnosed with ischaemic pain, AMI and unstable angina (196). Another study of 184 patients who presented to the ED with suspected cardiac chest pain showed that D-dimer levels taken at the time of presentation were on average 111% higher in patients who were diagnosed with ACS compared to those who were not. D-dimer (at a cut-off of 1mg/l) had a sensitivity of 18% in order to achieve a set specificity of

92%, although the implications of accepted a more conventional, lower D-dimer cut-off were not evaluated (197). In 102 patients who presented to a Brazilian ED, D-dimer levels at the time of ED presentation were significantly higher in patients who had a troponin T >0.01ng/ml at the time of presentation compared with patients whose troponin T was <0.01ng/ml. Unfortunately the results of 12-hour troponin testing were not available for analysis in this study, precluding evaluation of true diagnostic performance for AMI (198). The largest study to have investigated the use of D-dimer for the diagnosis of AMI in ED patients included a total of 741 patients who presented to the ED with suspected AMI. In that study, plasma D-dimer levels measured 12-24 hours after arrival at the ED had an AUC of 0.734 (95% CI 0.715 - 0.753) for predicting a troponin T result of >0.03ng/ml. At a cut-off of 500μg/l D-dimer had a sensitivity of 95%, specificity 27%, PPV 92% and NPV 41% (199). Finally, in a study of 432 patients who presented to the ED with suspected ACS D-dimer levels measured at the time of ED presentation did not help to predict the occurrence of adverse events (death, AMI, revascularisation, recurrent ACS or hospital admission with congestive heart failure) after 42 days of follow up (odds ratio 1.3, 95% CI 0.4 - 4.5, at a cut-off of 500μg/l).

The evidence suggests that D-dimer is unlikely to be useful as an early marker of AMI when used alone in the ED population and at present the evidence for the use of D-dimer as a prognostic marker is also sparse. Future research into this biomarker must focus upon evaluating its potential value as part of a multimarker strategy.

3.5 Markers of ventricular stress

3.5.1 Brain Natriuretic Peptide (BNP)

BNP was first isolated from porcine brains but it has since been recognised as a cardiac hormone synthesised predominantly by the ventricles in response to ventricular wall stress. Together with atrial natriuretic peptide, which is secreted primarily by the atria, BNP belongs to the natriuretic peptide family that is involved in cardiac homeostasis. Biological effects include diuresis, vasodilatation, inhibition of the renin-aldosterone system and of cardiac and vascular myocyte growth (200). BNP is known to be a marker of acute and chronic left ventricular dysfunction and may be useful for the ED diagnosis of the former (201,202). It has been used as a marker of left ventricular systolic dysfunction following AMI, where it provides prognostic information (203). BNP is also expressed in ischaemic human myocardium and plasma levels may rise during periods of ischaemia (204-208). A number of studies, that together have included a total of 5159 patients, have demonstrated that BNP level acts as a strong predictor of mortality at seven days, 30 days, six months and 10 months in patients with confirmed ACS (208-214). Other studies have shown that BNP levels help to predict all adverse cardiac events, both during the index hospital admission and at follow up after up to 1 year (215-217). BNP levels have also been shown to help predict the development of congestive heart failure when measured in patients with both STEMI and NSTE-ACS (218-219). In addition to having prognostic value, there is evidence that BNP may assist in the diagnosis of ACS. Several small case control studies have demonstrated higher BNP levels in patients with AMI (220-222) and unstable angina (223,224) when compared with controls. There is some evidence to suggest that BNP levels may, in fact, correlate with infarct size (225). However, among 1676 patients with confirmed NSTE-ACS only 15.6% of patients had BNP levels above 80pg/ml. Indeed only 25.2% of patients with NSTEMI had BNP levels above 80pg/ml, suggesting that BNP, at least at the stated diagnostic cut-off, may have limited sensitivity for these diagnoses (211).

In a study of 100 patients who were admitted to a Medical Admissions Unit with suspected cardiac chest pain, BNP (diagnostic cut-off 5pg/ml) helped to diagnose AMI with sensitivity 88.6%, specificity 78.6%, PPV 75%, NPV 89.6% with an AUC of 0.868. BNP was significantly more sensitive but less specific than troponin T when used at the time of admission to the unit. By combining BNP and troponin T performance improved (sensitivity 95.4%, specificity 76.8%). Unfortunately, however, this study had significant weaknesses as the primary outcome (discharge diagnosis of cardiac pain) could not be objectively verified through use of a gold standard, the study was retrospective and no follow up data was provided (226). Several studies have investigated the diagnostic and prognostic value of BNP levels in the ED population. Among 631 consecutive patients who presented to the ED with suspected cardiac chest pain with symptom onset <12 hours, BNP levels at the time of admission were found to be significantly higher among patients who were ultimately diagnosed with AMI (227). For predicting a diagnosis of AMI, BNP had an AUC of 0.710. Using a cut-off of 100pg/ml BNP predicted AMI with sensitivity 70.8%, specificity 68.9%, PPV 22.7%, NPV 94.8%, positive likelihood ratio 2.28 and negative likelihood ratio 0.42. When combined with CK-MB and troponin I, the presence of any raised biomarker for a diagnosis of AMI performed with sensitivity 87.3%, specificity 65.7%, PPV 27.0%, NPV 97.3%, positive likelihood ratio 2.55 and negative likelihood ratio 0.19. This suggests that, had BNP been introduced into clinical practice, this would have enabled the early detection of an additional 22 AMIs that could not otherwise have been recognised at the time of admission. However this would come at a cost of 163 false positive diagnoses (227). In a retrospective analysis of 546 patients who presented to the ED with suspected cardiac chest pain, a point-of-care BNP test was found to have an AUC of 0.755 for a diagnosis of AMI. At a cut-off of 100ng/l, BNP sensitivity was 66.7%, specificity 71.3%, PPV 17.1%, NPV 96.0%, positive likelihood ratio 2.32 and negative likelihood ratio 0.47. However the study had significant weaknesses. Clinicians were not blinded to BNP results, the study was subject to significant verification bias as only a minority of patients with normal point of care tests underwent subsequent gold standard troponin testing and, for those who did undergo troponin testing, an outdated troponin cut-off was used to diagnose AMI (228). Another study prospectively recruited 306 patients who presented to the ED with suspected cardiac chest pain. BNP was measured using two separate assays at the time of admission. The AUC of each assay for a diagnosis of ACS was found to be less than 0.6. BNP levels were found to be significant predictors of adverse events after 30 and 90 days but, again, the AUC was less than 0.7 for each assay (229).

Finally, in another prospective cohort study, 426 patients who presented to the ED with suspected cardiac chest pain had BNP levels measured at the time of presentation. The AUC of BNP for diagnosis of AMI, diagnosis of ACS and occurrence of adverse events (death, AMI or coronary revascularisation) within 30 days was 0.766, 0.691 and 0.675 respectively. The authors incorporated BNP into a multimarker strategy that also included CK-MB, myoglobin and troponin I. Using serial estimations at the time of ED presentation and 90 minutes later, this multimarker panel had a sensitivity of 97.4% (95% CI 86.5 - 100.0%), specificity 47.8% (42.7 - 52.9%), PPV 15.8% (11.5 - 21.1%) and NPV 99.5% (97.0 - 100.0%) for diagnosis of AMI. For a diagnosis of ACS performance was slightly worse, with a sensitivity of 88.1% and NPV 92.9% and for predicting adverse events within 30 days the panel performed with sensitivity 88.5%, specificity 43.9%, PPV 18.0% and NPV 96.5% (230). The available evidence suggests that BNP may have value as a diagnostic and prognostic marker in patients who present to the ED with suspected ACS. However it is readily apparent that BNP is unsuitable for use as a lone biomarker in this situation. Future research is still necessary in order to define the potential role of BNP as part of a multimarker strategy.

3.6 Novel markers of myocardial necrosis

3.6.1 Heart-type Fatty Acid Binding Protein (H-FABP)

H-FABP is a cytoplasmic protein that is abundantly expressed in human myocardial cells. It is also found in much lower concentration in skeletal muscle, kidney and brain tissue (231). Experimental data first suggested that H-FABP may be a potential novel biomarker of AMI as early as 1988 (232). In 1991 Tanaka et al reported elevated H-FABP levels in patients with AMI, with levels peaking earlier than CK-MB (233). Despite interest in H-FABP as an early marker of AMI for many years it has never gained widespread acceptance for use in clinical practice.

Five studies have investigated the diagnostic utility of H-FABP when used for the diagnosis of AMI at the time of presentation to the ED (234-238). Four of these studies utilised qualitative assays that are available as point of care tests. All five studies had significant weaknesses, with most studies employing now outdated gold standards for AMI diagnosis and being subject to significant verification bias. The data reporting in the small study by Alashemi et al precludes calculation of total sensitivity and specificity (235). If the remainder of the results are pooled this would give H-FABP a total sensitivity of 70.0% (95% CI 66.0 - 73.7%) and a total specificity of 80.7% (78.1 - 83.0). Excluding the study by Ghani et al, in which a quantitative assay was used, the pooled sensitivity is 76.8% (72.6 - 80.5%), pooled specificity 72.5% (68.9 - 75.8%), pooled PPV 65.8% (61.6 - 69.8%) and pooled NPV 82.0% (78.6 - 85.0%). The positive likelihood ratio would be 2.79 and negative likelihood ratio 0.32. It should be acknowledged that pooling results in this manner does not take account of heterogeneity and is inferior to a formal meta-analysis. However, assuming that these statistics are a true reflection of the performance of H-FABP, if we were to apply the test in a typical United Kingdom ED population with suspected cardiac chest pain who have a prevalence of AMI of approximately 18%, the post-test probability of AMI given a normal H-FABP test would be 6.6%. This provides similar predictive value to a normal ECG in this cohort (239) but is still far from excluding the diagnosis.

4. Multimarker strategy

Previous work from our own group, investigating heart fatty acid binding protein (H-FABP), CK-MB, myoglobin, cTnI, BNP, D-dimer, neutrophil gelatinase associated lipocalin (NGAL) and myeloperoxidase, in 705 patients presenting to the emergency department demonstrated that no single biomarker could exclude AMI. However multivariate analysis identified cTnI and H-FABP as an optimal biomarker combination. When combined with clinical risk stratification, the strategy exhibited a sensitivity of 96.9%, specificity of 54% and negative predictive value of 98%. [240].

The utility of a multimarker strategy must also be considered in the light of developments in assays. We have evaluated a high sensitivity troponin T assay in 915 patients, where the results demonstrated a negative predictive value of 99.4%. [241]

5. Conclusion

In recent years there has been substantial and growing interest in a number of novel biomarkers that may facilitate early diagnosis of AMI and enhanced risk stratification of patients who present to the ED with suspected ACS. Promising markers of each step in the pathophysiological evolution of an acute coronary syndrome have been identified, each of which may be detected in the peripheral circulation. Unfortunately it is unlikely that any of these biomarkers will be as cardio-specific as the cardiac troponins and, despite considerable research, there is at present no single biomarker that can be used to confirm or exclude a diagnosis of ACS in the ED. If there is to be a future for novel biomarkers in the ED diagnosis of ACS, therefore, future research must focus on incorporating levels of multiple biomarkers and available clinical information into a risk score or clinical decision rule, in order that the predictive value of individual biomarkers and clinical features may be combined and enhanced.

6. References

[1] British Heart Foundation. Mortality statistics 2004. www.heartstats.com . 2005. Ref Type: Generic

[2] Allender S, Peto V, Scarborough P, Boxer A, Rayner M. Coronary Heart Disease Statistics. 15th ed. London: British Heart Foundation; 2007.

[3] Fothergill NJ, Hunt MT, Touquet R. Audit of patients with chest pain presenting to an accident and emergency department over a 6-month period. Archives of Emergency Medicine 1993;10:155-60.

[4] Ekelund U, Nilsson HJ, Frigyesi A, Torffvit O. Patients with suspected acute coronary syndrome in a university hospital emergency department: an observational study. BMC Emergency Medicine 2002;2(1).

[5] Blatchford O, Capewell S, Murray S, Blatchford M. Emergency medical admission in Glasgow: general practices vary despite adjustment for age, sex and deprivation. British Journal of General Practice 1999;49:551-4.

[6] Collinson P, Premachandram S, Hashemi K. Prospective audit of incidence of prognostically important myocardial damage in patients discharged from emergency department. British Medical Journal 2000;320:1702-5.

[7] Pope JH, Aufderheide TP, Ruthazer R, Woolard RH, Feldman JA, Beshansky JR, et al. Missed diagnoses of acute cardiac ischaemia in the Emergency Department. N Engl J Med 2000;342:1163-70.

[8] Obrastzow WP, Straschesko ND. Zur Kenntnis der Thrombose der Koronararterien des Herzens. Z Klin Med 1910;71:116-32.

[9] Herrick JB. Clinical features of sudden obstruction of the coronary arteries. JAMA 1912;59:2015-20.

[10] Classics in arteriosclerosis research: an experimental cholesterin steatosis and its significance in the origin of some pathological processes by N. Anitschkow and S. Chalatow, translated by Mary Z. Pelias. Arteriosclerosis 1938;3:178-82.
[11] Stary HC, Chandler AB, Dinsmore RE, Fuster V, Glagov S, Insull W, et al. A definition of advanced types of atherosclerotic lesions and a histological classification of atherosclerosis. Circulation 1995;92:1355-74.
[12] Yokoya K, Takatsu H, Suzuki T, Hosokawa H, Ojio S, Matsubara T, et al. Process of progression of coronary artery lesions from mild or moderate stenosis to moderate or severe stenosis. A study based on four serial coronary arteriograms per year. Circulation 1999;100:903-9.
[13] Giroud D, Li JM, Urban P, Meier B, Rutishauser W. Relation of the site of acute myocardial infarction to the most severe coronary arterial stenosis at prior angiography. American Journal of Cardiology 1992;69:729-32.
[14] Little WC, Constantinescu M, Applegate RJ, Kutcher MA, Burrows MT, Kahl FR, et al. Can coronary angiography predict the site of subsequent myocardial infarction in patients with mild-to-moderate coronary artery disease? Circulation 1988;78:1157-66.
[15] Davies MJ. Stability and instability: two faces of coronary atherosclerosis. The Paul Dudley White Lecture 1995. Circulation 1996;94(8):2013-20.
[16] Kher N, Marsh JD. Pathobiology of atherosclerosis - a brief review. Seminars in Thrombosis and Haemostasis 2004;30(6):665-72.
[17] Libby P. Molecular bases of the acute coronary syndromes. Circulation 1995;91:2844-50.
[18] Glagov S, Weisenberd E, Zrins C, Stankunavicius R, Kolettis G. Compensatory enlargement of human atherosclerotic coronary arteries. New England Journal of Medicine 1987;316:1371-5.
[19] Ge J, Erbel R, Gerber T, Gorge G, Koch L, Haude M, et al. Intravascular ultrasound imaging of angiographically normal coronary arteries: a prospective study in vivo. British Heart Journal 1994;71(6):572-8.
[20] Ge J, Erbel R, Zamorano J, Koch L, Kearney P, Gorge G, et al. Coronary artery remodelling in atherosclerotic disease: an intravascular ultrasound study in vivo. Coronary Artery Disease 1993;4:981-6.
[21] Losordo DW, Rosenfield K, Kaufman J, Pieczek A, Isner JM. Focal compensatory enlargement of human arteries in response to progressive atherosclerosis: in vivo documentation using intravascular ultrasound. Circulation 1994;89:2570-7.
[22] Libby P, Ridker PM. Inflammation and atherothrombosis: From population biology and bench research to clinical practice. Journal of the American College of Cardiology 2006;48(9 Suppl A):33-46.
[23] Szmitko PE, Wang CH, Weisel RD, de Almeida JR, Anderson TJ, Verma S. New markers of inflammation and endothelial cell activation Part 1. Circulation 2003;108:1917-23.
[24] Szmitko PE, Wang CH, Weisel RD, Jeffries GA, Anderson TJ, Verma S. Biomarkers of vascular disease linking inflammation to endothelial activation. Part 2. Circulation 2003;108(17):2041-8.
[25] Libby P, Ridker PM, Maseri A. Inflammation and atherosclerosis. Circulation 2002;105:1135-43.

[26] Behrendt D, Ganz P. Endothelial function: from vascular biology to clinical applications. American Journal of Cardiology 2002;90(Suppl):40L-8L.
[27] Ross R. Atherosclerosis - an inflammatory disease. N Engl J Med 1999;340(2):115-26.
[28] Hoppeler H, Kayar SR. Capillarity and oxidative capacity of muscle. News in Physiolical Science 1988;3:113-6.
[29] Bevilacqua MP. Endothelial-leukocyte adhesion molecules. Annual Reviews of Immunology 1993;11:767-804.
[30] Weissman G. The role of neutrophils in vascular injury: a summary of signal transduction mechanisms in cell/cell interactions. Springer Seminars in Immunopathology 1989;11:235-58.
[31] Gauthier TW, Scalia R, Murohara T, Guo JP, Lefer AM. Nitric oxide protects against leukocyte-endothelium interactions in the early stages of hypercholesterolaemia. Arteriosclerosis, Thrombosis & Vascular Biology 1995;15:1652-9.
[32] Kubes P, Suzuki M, Granger DN. Nitric oxide: an endogenous modulator of leukocyte adhesion. Proceedings of the National Academy of Sciences USA 1991;88:4651-5.
[33] Cornwell TL, Arnold E, Boerth NJ, Lincoln TM. Inhibition of smooth muscle cell growth by nitric oxide and activation of cAMP-dependent protein kinase by cGMP. American Journal of Physiology 1994;267:C1405-C1413.
[34] de Graaf JC, Banga JD, Moncada S, Palmer RM, de Groot PG, Sixma JJ. Nitric oxide functions as an inhibitor of platelet adhesion under flow conditions. Circulation 1992;85:2284-90.
[35] Springer TA. Traffic signals for lymphocyte recirculation and leukocyte emigration: the multistep paradigm. Cell 1994;76:301-14.
[36] Adams DH, Lloyd AR. Chemokines: leukocyte recruitment and activation cytokines. Lancet 1997;349:490-5.
[37] Gearing AJH, Newman W. Circulating adhesion molecules in disease. Immunology Today 1993;14(10):506-12.
[38] Price DT, Loscalzo J. Cellular adhesion molecules and atherogenesis. American Journal of Medicine 1999;107:85-97.
[39] Tiong AY, Brieger D. Inflammation and coronary artery disease. American Heart Journal 2005;150(1):11-8.
[40] Podrez EA, Febbraio M, Sheibani N, Schmitt D, Silberstein RL, Hajjar DP, et al. Macrophage scavenger receptor CD36 is the major receptor for LDL modified by monocyte-generated reactive nitrogen species. Journal of Clinical Investigation 2000;105:1095-108.
[41] Podrez EA, Schmitt D, Hoff HF, Hazen SL. Myeloperoxidase-generated reactive nitrogen species convert LDL into an atherogenic form in vivo. Journal of Clinical Investigation 1999;103:1547-60.
[42] Fu X, Kassim SY, Parks WC, Heinecke JW. Hypochlorous acid oxygenates the cysteine switch domain of pro-matrilysn (MMP-7). J Biol Chem 2001;276(44):41279-87.
[43] Sugiyama S, Okada Y, Sukhova GK, Virmani R, Heinecke JW, Libby P. Macrophage myeloperoxidase regulation by granulocyte macrophage colony-stimulating factor in human atherosclerosis and implications in acute coronary syndromes. American Journal of Pathology 2001;158(3):879-91.

[44] Schonbeck U, Libby P. The CD40/CD154 receptor/ligand dyad. Cellular and Molecular Life Sciences 2001;58:4-43.

[45] Mach F, Schonbeck U, Sukhova GK, Bourcier T, Bonnefoy JY, Pober JS, et al. Functional CD40 ligand is expressed on human vascular endothelial cells, smooth muscle cells, and macrophages: Implications for CD40-CD40 ligand signaling in atherosclerosis. PNAS 1997 Mar 4;94(5):1931-6.

[46] Urbich C, Dernbach E, Aicher A, Zeiher AM, Dimmeler S. CD40 ligand inhibits endothelial cell migration by increasing production of endothelial reactive oxygen species. Circulation 2002;106:981-6.

[47] Schonbeck U, Sukhova GK, Shimizu K, Mach F, Libby P. Inhibition of CD40 signalling limits evolution of established atherosclerosis in mice. PNAS 2000;97(13):7458-63.

[48] Peng DQ, Zhao SP, Li YF, Li J, Zhou HN. Elevated soluble CD40 ligand is related to the endothelial adhesion molecules in patients with acute coronary syndromes. Clinica Chimica Acta 2002;319:19-26.

[49] Schonbeck U, Libby P. CD40 signaling and plaque instability. Circulation Research 2001;89:1092-103.

[50] Lindmark E, Tenno T, Siegbahn A. Role of platelet P-selectin and CD40 ligand in the induction of monocytic tissue factor expression. Arteriosclerosis, Thrombosis & Vascular Biology 2000;20:2322-8.

[51] Geng YJ, Libby P. Progression of atheroma: a struggle between death and procreation. Arteriosclerosis, Thrombosis & Vascular Biology 2002;22:1370-80.

[52] van Zanten GH, de Graaf S, Slootweg PJ, Heijnen HFG, Connolly TM, de Groot PG, et al. Increased platelet deposition on atherosclerotic coronary arteries. Journal of Clinical Investigation 1994;93:615-32.

[53] van der Wal AC, Becker AE, van der Loos CM, Das PK. Site of intimal rupture or erosion of thrombosed coronary atherosclerotic plaques is characterized by an inflammatory process irrespective of the dominant plaque morphology. Circulation 1994;89:36-44.

[54] Bayes-Genis A, Conover CA, Overgaard MT, Bailey KR, Christiansen M, Holmes DR, et al. Pregnancy-associated plasma protein A as a marker of acute coronary syndromes. New England Journal of Medicine 2001;345(14):1022-9.

[55] Virmani R, Burke AP, Farb A, Kolodgie FD. Pathology of the vulnerable plaque. Journal of the American College of Cardiology 2006;47:C13-C18.

[56] Davies MJ. A macro and micro view of coronary vascular insult in ischemic heart disease. Circulation 1990;82(Suppl 1):I-1138-I-1146.

[57] Farb A, Burke AP, Tang AL, Liang Y, Mannan P, Smialek J, et al. Coronary plaque erosion without rupture into a lipid core: a frequent cause of coronary thrombosis in sudden coronary death. Circulation 1996;93:1354-63.

[58] Cheng G, Loree H, Kamm R, Fishbein M, Lee R. Distribution of circumferential stress in ruptured and stable atherosclerotic lesions: a structural analysis with histopathological correlation. Circulation 1993;87:1179-87.

[59] Richardson P, Davies M, Born G. Influence of plaque configuration and stress distribution on fissuring of coronary atherosclerotic plaques. Lancet 1989;334(8669):941-4.

[60] Muller JE, Abela GS, Nesto RW, Tofler GH. Triggers, acute risk factors and vulnerable plaques: the lexicon of a new frontier. Journal of the American College of Cardiology 1994;23:809-13.
[61] Shah PK. Plaque disruption and coronary thrombosis: new insight into pathogenesis and prevention. Clin Cardiol 1997;20(Suppl II):II-38-II-44.
[62] Andre P, Prasad S, Denis CV, He M, Papalia JM, Hynes RO, et al. CD40L stabilizes arterial thrombi by a beta3 integrin-dependent mechanism. Nature Medicine 2002;8(3):247-52.
[63] Merten M, Chow T, Hellums JD, Thiagarajan P. A New Role for P-Selectin in Shear-Induced Platelet Aggregation. Circulation 2000;102(17):2045-50.
[64] Merten M, Thiagarajan P. P-Selectin Expression on Platelets Determines Size and Stability of Platelet Aggregates. Circulation 2000;102(16):1931-6.
[65] Blann AD, Nadar SK, Lip GYH. The adhesion molecule P-selectin and cardiovascular disease. European Heart Journal 2003;24:2166-79.
[66] Viallard JF, Solanilla A, Gauthier B, Contin C, Dechanet J, Grosset C, et al. Increased soluble and platelet-associated CD40 ligand in essential thrombocythemia and reactive thrombocytosis. Blood 2002;99:2612-4.
[67] Davies M, Bland J, Hangartner J, Angelini A, Thomas A. Factors influencing the presence or absence of acute coronary artery thrombi in sudden ischemic death. European Heart Journal 1989;10:203-8.
[68] Davies M, Thomas A. Thrombosis and acute coronary artery lesions in sudden cardiac ischemic death. New England Journal of Medicine 1984;310:1137-40.
[69] Frink R. Chronic ulcerated plaques: new insights into the pathogenesis of acute coronary disease. Journal of Invasive Cardiology 1994;6:173-85.
[70] Falk E. Plaque rupture with severe pre-existing stenosis precipitating coronary thrombosis. British Heart Journal 1983;1983(50):-127.
[71] Willerson JTGP, Eidt J, Campbell WB, Buja M. Specific platelet mediators and unstable coronary artery lesions: experimental evidence and potential clinical imlications. Circulation 1989;80:198-205.
[72] Ferguson JL, Beckett GJ, Stoddart M, Walker SW, Fox KAA. Myocardial infarction redefined: the new ACC/ESC definition, based on cardiac troponin, increases the apparent incidence of infarction. Heart 2002;88:343-7.
[73] Johnson-Tidey RR, McGregor JL, Taylor PR, Poston RN. Increase in the adhesion molecule P-selectin in endothelium overlying atherosclerotic plaques. American Journal of Pathology 1994;144(5):952-61.
[74] Koyama H, Maeno T, Fukumoto S, Shoji T, Yamane T, Yokoyama H, et al. Platelet P-selectin expression is associated with atherosclerotic wall thickness in carotid artery in humans. Circulation 2003;2003(108):-524.
[75] Tenaglia AN, Buda AJ, Wilkins RG, et al. Levels of expression of P-selectin, E-selectin and inter cellular adhesion molecule-1 in coronary atherectomy specimens from patients with stable and unstable angina pectoris. American Journal of Cardiology 1997;79:742-7.
[76] Hsu-Lin S, Berman CL, Furie BC, August D, Furie B. A platelet membrane protein expressed during platelet activation and secretion. Studies using a monoclonal antibody specific for thrombin- activated platelets. J Biol Chem 1984;259(14):9121-6.

[77] Shimomura H, Ogawa H, Arai H, Moriyama Y, Takazoe K, Hirai N, et al. Serial changes in plasma levels of soluble P-selectin in patients with acute myocardial infarction. American Journal of Cardiology 1998;81:397-400.
[78] Ikeda H, Nakayama H, Oda T, Kuwano K, Muraishi A, Sugi K, et al. Soluble form of P-selectin in patients with acute myocardial infarction. Coronary Artery Disease 1994;5(6):515-8.
[79] Gurbel PA, O'Connor CM, Dalesandro MR, Serebruany VL. Relation of soluble and platelet P-selectin to early outcome in patients with acute myocardial infarction after thrombolytic therapy. American Journal of Cardiology 2001;87(15):774-7.
[80] Mulvihill NT, Foley JB, Murphy R, Crean P, Walsh M. Evidence of prolonged inflammation in unstable angina and non-Q wave myocardial infarction. Journal of the American College of Cardiology 2000;36(4):1210-6.
[81] Xu DY, Zhao SP, Peng WP. Elevated plasma levels of soluble P-selectin in patients with acute myocardial infarction and unstable angina: An inverse link to lipoprotein(a). International Journal of Cardiology 1998;64:253-8.
[82] Guray U, Erbay AR, Guray Y, Yilmaz B, Boyaci AA, Sasmaz H, et al. Levels of soluble adhesion molecules in various clinical presentations of coronary atherosclerosis. International Journal of Cardiology 2004;96:235-40.
[83] Chiu CA, Wu CJ, Yang CH, Fang CY, Hsieh YK, Hang CL, et al. Levels and value of soluble P-selectin following acute myocardial infarction: evaluating the link between soluble P-selectin levels and recruitment of circulating white blood cells and the marker for the rapid diagnosis of chest pain. Chang Gung Medical Journal 28(10):699-707, 2005.
[84] Liu WH, Yang CH, Yeh KH, Chang HW, Chen YH, Chen SM, et al. Circulating levels of soluble P-selectin in patients in the early and recent phases of myocardial infarction. Chang Gung Medical Journal 28(9):613-20, 2005.
[85] Atalar E, Aytemir K, Haznedaroglu I, Ozer N, Ovunc K, Aksoyek S, et al. Increased plasma levels of soluble selectins in patients with unstable angina. International Journal of Cardiology 2001;78:69-73.
[86] Ikeda H, TAkajo Y, Ichiki K, Ueno T, Maki S, Noda T, et al. Increased soluble form of P-selectin in patients with unstable angina. Circulation 1995;92:1693-6.
[87] Parker C 3rd, Vita JA, Freedman JE. Soluble adhesion molecules and unstable coronary artery disease. Atherosclerosis 2001;156(2):417-24.
[88] Venturinelli ML, Hovnan A, Soeiro AM, Nicolau JC, Ramires JA, D'Amico EA, et al. Platelet activation in different clinical forms of the coronary artery disease (role of P-selectin and others platelet markers in stable and unstable angina). Arquivos Brasileiros de Cardiologia 2006;87(4):446-50.
[89] Ault KA, Cannon CP, Mitchell J, McCahan J, Tracy RP, Novotny WF, et al. Platelet activation in patients after an acute coronary syndrome: Results from the TIMI-12 trial. Journal of the American College of Cardiology 1999;33:634-9.
[90] Itoh T, Nakai K, Ono M, Hiramori K. Can the risk for acute cardiac events in acute coronary syndrome be indicated by platelet membrane activation marker P-selectin? Coronary Artery Disease 1995;6(8):645-50.

[91] Mulvihill NT, Foley JB, Murphy RT, Curtin R, Crean PA, Walsh M. Risk stratification in unstable angina and non-q wave myocardial infarction using soluble cell adhesion molecules. Heart 2001;85:623-7.
[92] Soeki T, Tamura Y, Shinohara H, Sakabe K, Onose Y, Fukuda N. Increased soluble platelet/endothelial cell adhesion molecule-1 in the early stages of acute coronary syndromes. International Journal of Cardiology 2003;90:261-8.
[93] Kavsak PA, Ko DT, Newman AM, Lustig V, Palomaki GE, Macrae AR, et al. Vascular versus myocardial dysfunction in acute coronary syndrome: Are the adhesion molecules as powerful as NT-proBNP for long-term risk stratification? Clinical Biochemistry 2008;6:436-9.
[94] Serebruany VL, Murugesan SR, Pothula A, Semaan H, Gurbel PA. Soluble PECAM-1, but not P-selectin, nor osteonectin identify acute myocardial infarction in patients presenting with chest pain. Cardiology 1999;91(1):50-5.
[95] Serebruany VL, Levine DJ, Nair GV, Meister AF, Gurbel PA. Usefulness of combining necrosis and platelet markeres in triaging patients presenting with chest pain to the Emergency Department. Journal of Thrombosis and Thrombolysis 2001;11:155-62.
[96] Hillis GS, Terregino C, Taggart P, Killian A, Zhao N, Dalsey WC, et al. Elevated soluble P-selectin levels are associated with an increased risk of early adverse events in patients with presumed myocardial ischemia. American Heart Journal 2002;143:235-41.
[97] Hollander JE, Muttreja R, Dalesandro MR, Shofer FS. Risk stratification of emergency patients with acute coronary syndromes using P-selectin. Journal of the American College of Cardiology 1999;34:95-105.
[98] Gurbel PA, Kereiakes DJ, Dalesandro MR, et al. Role of soluble and platelet bound P-selectin in discriminating cardiac from non cardiac chest pain at presentation in the emergency department. American Heart Journal 2000;139:320-8.
[99] R, Pemberton P, Ali F et al. Low soluble P-selectin may facilitate early exclusion of acute myocardial infarction. Clin Chem Acta 2011; 412: 614-8
[100] Oishi Y, Wakatsuki T, Nishikado A, Oki T, Ito S. Circulating adhesion molecules and severity of coronary atherosclerosis. Coronary Artery Disease 2000;11(1):77-81.
[101] Squadrito F, Altavilla D, Ioculano M, Canale P, Campo GM, Squadrito G, et al. Soluble E-selectin levels in acute human myocardial infarction. International Journal of Microcirculation: Clinical & Experimental 1995;15(2):80-4.
[102] Miyao Y, Miyazaki S, Goto Y, Itoh A, Daikoku S, Morli I, et al. Role of cytokines and adhesion molecules in ischemia and reperfusion in patients with acute myocardial infarction. Japanese Circulation Journal 1999;63(5):362-5.
[103] Zeitler H, Ko Y, Zimmerman C, Nickenig G, Glanzer K, Walger P, et al. Elevated serum concentrations of soluble adhesion molecules in coronary artery disease and acute myocardial infarction. European Journal of Medical Research 1997;2(9):389-94.
[104] Li YH, Teng JK, Tsai WC, Lin LJ, Chen JH. Elevated levels of soluble adhesion molecules is associated with the severity of myocardial damage in acute myocardial infarction. American Journal of Cardiology 1997;80:1218-21.
[105] Suefuji H, Ogawa H, Yasue H, Sakamoto T, Miyao Y, Kaikita K, et al. Increased plasma level of soluble E-selectin in acute myocardial infarction. American Heart Journal 2000;140:243-8.

[106] Pellegatta F, Pizzetti G, Lu Y, Radaelli A, Pomes D, Carlino M, et al. Soluble E-selectin and intercellular adhesion molecule-1 plasma levels increase during acute myocardial infaction. J Cardiovasc Pharmacol 1997;30(4):455-60.
[107] Siminiak T, Dye JF, Egdell RM, More R, Wysocki H, Sheridan DJ. The release of soluble adhesion molecules ICAM-1 and E-selectin after acute myocardial infarction and following coronary angioplasty. International Journal of Cardiology 1997;61(2):113-8.
[108] Squadrito F, Saitta A, Altavilla D, Ioculano M, Canale P, Campo GM, et al. Thrombolytic therapy with urokinase reduces increased circulating endothelial adhesion molecules in acute myocardial infarction. Inflammation Research 1996;45(1):14-9.
[109] Ghaisas NK, Shahi CN, Foley B, Goggins M, Crean P, Kelly A, et al. Elevated levels of circulating soluble adhesion molecules in peripheral blood of patients with unstable angina. American Journal of Cardiology 1997;80:617-9.
[110] Xie Y, Zhou T, Shen W, Lu G, Yin T, Gong L. Soluble cell adhesion molecules in patients with acute coronary syndrome. Chinese Medical Journal 2000;113(3):286-8.
[111] Mulvihill N, Foley JB, Ghaisas N, Murphy R, Crean P, Walsh M. Early temporal expression of soluble cellular adhesion molecules in patients with unstable angina and subendocardial myocardial infarction. American Journal of Cardiology 1999;83:1265-7.
[112] Boos CJ, Balakrishnan B, Blann AD, Lip GYH. The relationship of circulating endothelial cells to plasma indices of endothelial damage/dysfunction and apoptosis in acute coronary syndromes: Implications for prognosis. Journal of Thrombosis and Haemostasis 2008;6(11):1841-50.
[113] Miwa K, Igawa A, Inoue H. Soluble E-selectin, ICAM-1 and VCAM-1 levels in systemic and coronary circulation in patients with variant angina. Cardiovascular Research 1997;36(1):37-44.
[114] Siminiak T, Smielecki J, Dye JF, Balinski M, El-Gendi H, Wysocki H, et al. Increased release of the soluble form of the adhesion molecules L-selectin and ICAM-1 but not E-selectin during attacks of angina pectoris. Heart & Vessels 1998;13(4):189-94.
[115] Gurbel PA, Serebruany VL. Soluble vascular cell adhesion molecule-1 and E-selectin in patients with acute myocardial infarction treated with thrombolytic agents. American Journal of Cardiology 1998;81:772-5.
[116] Galvani M, Ferrini D, Ottani F, Nanni C, Ramberti A, Amboni P, et al. Soluble E-selectin is not a marker of unstable coronary plaque in serum of patients with ischemic heart disease. Journal of Thrombosis & Thrombolysis 2000;9(1):53-60.
[117] Shyu KG, Chang H, Lin CC, Kuan P. Circulating intercellular adhesion molecule-1 and E-selectin in patients with acute coronary syndrome. Chest 1996;109:1627-30.
[118] Hope SA, Meredith IT, Farouque HMO, Worthley SG, Plunkett JC, Balazs ND. Time course of plasma adhesion molecules in acute coronary syndromes. Coronary Artery Disease 2002;13:215-21.
[119] Ridker PM, Hennekens CH, Roitman-Johnson B, Stampfer MJ, Allen J. Plasma concentration of soluble intercellular adhesion molecule-1 and risks of future myocardial infarction in apparently healthy men. Lancet 1998;351:88-92.

[120] Luc G, Arveiler D, Evans A, Amouyel P, Ferrieres J, Bard MJ, et al. Circulating soluble adhesion molecules ICAM-1 and VCAM-1 and incident coronary heart disease: The PRIME Study. Atherosclerosis 2003;170:169-76.
[121] Empana J-P, Canoui-Poitrine F, Luc G, Juhan-Vague I, Morange P, Arveiler D, et al. Contribution of novel biomarkers to incident stable angina and acute coronary syndrome: The PRIME Study. European Heart Journal 2008;29(16):1966-74.
[122] Ridker PM, Hennekens CH, Buring JE, Rifai N. C-reactive protein and other markers of inflammation in the prediction of cardiovascular disease in women. New England Journal of Medicine 2000;3442:836-43.
[123] Shai I, Pischon T, Hu FB, Ascherio A, Rifai N, Rimm EB. Soluble intercellular adhesion molecules, soluble vascular cell adhesion molecules, and risk of coronary heart disease. Obesity 2006;14(11):2099-106.
[124] Albert MA, Glynn RJ, Buring JE, Ridker PM. Differential effect of soluble intercellular adhesion molecule-1 on the progression of atherosclerosis as compared to arterial thrombosis: a prospective analysis of the Women's Health Study. Atherosclerosis 1997;(1):297-302.
[125] Morisaki N, Saito I, Tamura K, Tashiro J, Masuda M, Kanzaki T, et al. New indices of ischemic heart disease and aging: studies on the serum levels of soluble intercellular adhesion molecule-1 (ICAM-1) and soluble vascular cell adhesion molecules-1 (VCAM-1) in patients with hypercholesterolemia and ischemic heart disease. Atherosclerosis 1997;131:43-8.
[126] Haim M, Tanne D, Boyko V, Reshef T, Goldbourt U, Leor J, et al. Soluble intercellular adhesion molecule-1 and long-term risk of acute coronary events in patients with coronary heart disease. Journal of the American College of Cardiology 2002;39(7):1133-8.
[127] Wallen NH, Held C, Rehnqvist N, Hjemdahl P. Elevated serum intercellular adhesion molecule-1 and vascular adhesion molecule-1 among patients with stable angina pectoris who suffer cardiovascular death or non-fatal myocardial infarction. European Heart Journal 1999;20:1039-43.
[128] Postadzhiyan AS, Tzontcheva AV, Kehayov I, Finkov B. Circulating soluble adhesion molecules ICAM-1 and VCAM-1 and their association with clinical outcome, troponin T and C-reactive protein in patients with acute coronary syndromes. Clinical Biochemistry 2008;41(3):126-33.
[129] Tousoulis D, Antoniades C, Bosinakou E, Kotsopoulou M, Tsoufis C, Marinou K, et al. Differences in inflammatory and thrombotic markers between unstable angina and acute myocardial infarction. International Journal of Cardiology 115(2):203-7, 2007 Feb 7.
[130] Tekin G, Tekin A, Sipahi I, Kaya A, Sansoy V. Plasma concentration of soluble vascular cell adhesion molecule-1 and oncoming cardiovascular risk in patients with unstable angina pectoris and non-ST-segment elevation myocardial infarction. American Journal of Cardiology 2005;96(3):379-81.
[131] Chen WQ, Zhang M, Ji XP, Ding SF, Zhao YX, Chen YG, et al. Usefulness of high-frequency vascular ultrasound imaging and serum inflammatory markers to predict plaque rupture in patients with stable and unstable angina pectoris. American Journal of Cardiology 2007;100(9):1341-6.

[132] Hartford M, Wiklund O, Mattsson HL, Persson A, Karlsson T, Herlitz J, et al. C-reactive protein, interleukin-6, secretory phospholipase A2 group IIA and intercellular adhesion molecule-1 in the prediction of late outcome events after acute coronary syndromes. Journal of Internal Medicine 2007;262(5):526-36.
[133] Rallidis LS, Gika HI, Zolindaki MG, Xydas TA, Paravolidakis KE. Usefulness of elevated levels of soluble vascular cell adhesion molecule-1 in predicting in-hospital prognosis in patients with unstable angina pectoris. American Journal of Cardiology 2003;92(10):1195-7.
[134] Murphy RT, Foley JB, Mulvihill N, Crean P, Walsh MJ. Endothelial inflammation and thrombolysis resistance in acute myocardial infarction. International Journal of Cardiology 2002;83:227-31.
[135] Parissis JT, Adamopoulous S, Venetsanou K, Kostakis G, Rigas A, Karas SM, et al. Plasma profiles of circulating granulocyte-macrophages colony-stimulating factor and soluble cellular adhesion molecules in acute myocardial infarction. Contribution to post-infarction left ventricular dysfunction. European Cytokine Network 2004;15(2):139-44.
[136] Murohara T, Kamijikkoku S, Honda T. Increased circulating soluble intercellular adhesion molecule-1 in acute myocardial infarction: A possible predictor of reperfusion ventricular arrhythmias. Critical Care Medicine 2000;28(6):1861-4.
[137] Kamijikkoku S, Murohara T, Tayama S, Matsuyama K, Honda T, Ando M, et al. Acute myocardial infarction and increased soluble intercellular adhesion molecule-1: A marker of vascular inflammation and a risk of early restenosis? American Heart Journal 1998;136(2):231-6.
[138] O'Malley TO, Ludlam CA, Tiemermsa RA, Fox KAA. Early increase in levels of soluble inter-cellular adhesion molecule-1 (sICAM-1). Potential risk factor for the acute coronary syndromes. European Heart Journal 2001;22:1226-34.
[139] Menown IBA, Mathew TP, Gracey HM, Nesbitt GS, Murray P, Young IS, et al. Prediction of recurrent events by D-dimer and inflammatory markers in patients with normal cardiac troponin I (PREDICT Study). American Heart Journal 2003;145:986-92.
[140] Hillis GS, Terregino C, Taggart P, Killian A, Zhao N, Kaplan J, et al. Soluble intercellular adhesion molecule-1 as a predictor of early adverse events in patients with chest pain compatible with myocardial ischemia. Annals of Emergency Medicine 2001;38(3):223-8.
[141] Heeschen C, Dimmeler S, Hamm CW, Van den Brand MJ, Boersma E, Zeiher AM, et al. Soluble CD40 ligand in acute coronary syndromes. New England Journal of Medicine 2003;348:1104-11.
[142] Aukrust P, Muller F, Ueland T, Berget T, Aeser E, Brunsvig A, et al. Enhanced levels of soluble and membrane-bound CD40 ligand in patients with unstable angina. Possible reflection of T lymphocyte and platelet involvement in the pathogenesis of acute coronary syndromes. Circulation 1999;100(6):614-20.
[143] Garlichs CD, Eskafi S, Raaz D, Schmitdt A, Ludwig J, Herrmann M, et al. Patients with acute coronary syndromes express enhanced CD40 ligand/CD154 on platelets. Heart 2001;86:649-55.

[144] Yan J, Wu Z, Huang Z, Li L, Zhong R, Kong X. Clinical implications of increased expression of CD40L in patients with acute coronary syndromes. Chinese Medical Journal 2002;115(4):491-3.
[145] Varo N, de Lemos JA, Libby P, Morrow DA, Murphy SA, Nuzzo R, et al. Soluble CD40L. Risk prediction after acute coronary syndromes. Circulation 2003;108:1049-52.
[146] Yan JC, Wu ZG, ?Kong XT, Zong RQ, Zhan LZ. Relation between upregulation of CD40 system and complex stenosis morphology in patients with acute coronary syndrome. Acta Pharmacologica Sinica 2004;25(2):251-6.
[147] Yan JC, Zhu J, Gao L, Wu ZG, Kong XT, Zong RQ, et al. The effect of elevated serum soluble CD40 ligand on the prognostic value in patients with acute coronary syndromes. Clinica Chimica Acta 2004;343:155-9.
[148] Tousoulis D, Antoniades C, Nikolopoulou A, Koniari K, Vasiliadou C, Marinou K, et al. Interaction between cytokines and sCD40L in patients with stable and unstable coronary syndromes. European Journal of Clinical Investigation 2007;37(8):623-8.
[149] Malarstig A, Lindahl B, Wallentin L, Siegbahn A. Soluble CD40L levels are regulated by the -3459 A>G polymorphism and predict myocardial infarction and the efficacy of antithrombotic treatment in non-ST elevation acute coronary syndrome. Arteriosclerosis, Thrombosis & Vascular Biology 2006;26(7):1667-73.
[150] Yip HK, Wu CJ, Yang CH, Chang HW, Fang CY, Hung WC, et al. Serial changes in circulating concentrations of soluble CD40 ligand and C-reactive protein in patients with unstable angina undergoing coronary stenting. Circulation Journal 2005;69(8):890-5.
[151] Tan J, Hua Q, Gao J, Zhen XF. Clinical implications of elevated serum interleukin-6, soluble CD40 ligand, metalloproteinase-9, and tissue inhibitor of metalloproteinase-1 in patients with acute ST-segment elevation myocardial infarction. Clinical Cardiology 2008;31(9):413-8.
[152] Dominguez-Rodriguez A, breu-Gonzalez P, Garcia-Gonzalez MJ, Kaski JC. Soluble CD40 ligand:interleukin-10 ratio predicts in-hospital adverse events in patients with ST-segment elevation myocardial infarction.[see comment]. Thrombosis Research 121(3):293-9, 2007.
[153] Apple FS, Pearce LA, Chung A, Ler R, Murakami MM. Multiple biomarker use for detection of adverse events in patients presenting with symptoms suggestive of acute coronary syndrome. Clinical Chemistry 2007;53(5):874-81.
[154] Brugger-Andersen T, Aarsetoy H, Grundt H, Staines H, Nilsen DWT. The long-term prognostic value of multiple biomarkers following a myocardial infarction. Thrombosis Research 2008;123(1):60-6.
[155] Abu-Soud HM, Hazen SL. Nitric oxide is a physiological substrate for mammalian peroxidases. J Biol Chem 2000;275(48):37524-32.
[156] Podrez EA, Poliakov E, Shen Z, Zhang R, Deng Y, Sun M, et al. A novel family of atherogenic oxidized phospholipids promotes macrophage foam cell formation via the scavenber receptor CD36 and is enriched in atherosclerotic lesions. J Biol Chem 2002;277(41):38517-23.
[157] Biasucci LM, D'Onofrio G, Liuzzo G, Zini G, Monaco C, Caligiuri G, et al. Intracellular neutrophil myeloperoxidase is reduced in unstable angina and acute myocardial

infarction, but its reduction is not related to ischemia. Journal of the American College of Cardiology 1996;27(3):611-6.

[158] Zhang R, Brennan ML, Fu X, Aviles RJ, Pearce GL, Penn MS, et al. Association between myeloperoxidase levels and risk of coronary artery disease. JAMA 2001;2886:2136-42.

[159] Ndrepepa G, Braun S, Mehilli J, von BN, Schomig A, Kastrati A. Myeloperoxidase level in patients with stable coronary artery disease and acute coronary syndromes. European Journal of Clinical Investigation 2008;38(2):90-6.

[160] Baldus S, Heeschen C, Meinertz T, Zeiher AM, Eiserich JP, Munzel T, et al. Myeloperoxidase serum levels predict risk in patients with acute coronary syndromes. Circulation 2003;108:1440-5.

[161] Morrow DA, Sabatine MS, Brennan ML, de Lemos JA, Murphy SA, Ruff CT, et al. Concurrent evaluation of novel cardiac biomarkers in acute coronary syndrome: myeloperoxidase and soluble CD40 ligand and the risk of recurrent ischaemic events in TACTICS-TIMI 18. European Heart Journal 2008;29(9):1096-102.

[162] Khan SQ, Kelly D, Quinn P, Davies JE, Ng LL. Myeloperoxidase aids prognostication together with N-terminal pro-B-type natriuretic peptide in high-risk patients with acute ST elevation myocardial infarction. Heart 2007;93(7):826-31.

[163] Mocatta TJ, Pilbrow AP, Cameron VA, Senthilmohan R, Frampton CM, Richards AM, et al. Plasma concentrations of myeloperoxidase predict mortality after myocardial infarction.[see comment]. Journal of the American College of Cardiology 2007;49(20):1993-2000.

[164] Cavusoglu E, Ruwende C, Eng C, Chopra V, Yanamadala S, Clark LT, et al. Usefulness of baseline plasma myeloperoxidase levels as an independent predictor of myocardial infarction at two years in patients presenting with acute coronary syndrome. American Journal of Cardiology 2007;99(10):1364-8.

[165] Wang J, Xing Y, Ma C, Li S, Li Z, Gao Y, et al. Clinical correlation between myeloperoxidase and acute coronary syndrome. Journal of Geriatric Cardiology 2007;4(4):209-12.

[166] Cavusoglu E, Ruwende C, Chopra V, Yanamadala S, Eng C, Clark LT, et al. Adiponectin is an independent predictor of all-cause mortality, cardiac mortality, and myocardial infarction in patients presenting with chest pain.[see comment]. European Heart Journal 2006;27(19):2300-9.

[167] Brennan ML, Penn MS, Van Lente F, Nambi V, Shishenbor MH, Aviles RJ, et al. Prognostic value of myeloperoxidase in patients with chest pain. New England Journal of Medicine 2003;349:1595-604.

[168] Mitchell AM, Garvey JL, Kline JA. Multimarker panel to rule out acute coronary syndromes in low-risk patients. Academic Emergency Medicine 13(7):803-6, 2006 Jul.

[169] Esporcatte R, Rey HC, Rangel FO, Rocha RM, Mendonca Filho HT, Dohmann HF, et al. Predictive value of myeloperoxidase to identify high risk patients admitted to the hospital with acute chest pain. Arquivos Brasileiros de Cardiologia 2007;89(6):377-84.

[170] Newby AC. Dual role of matrix metalloproteinases (matrixins) in intimal thickening and atherosclerotic plaque rupture. Physiology Reviews 2005;85:1-31.

[171] Henney AM, Wakeley PR, Davies MJ, Foster K, Hembry R, Murphy G, et al. Localization of Stromelysin Gene Expression in Atherosclerotic Plaques by in situ Hybridization. PNAS 1991 Sep 15;88(18):8154-8.
[172] Galis ZS, Sukhova GK, Lark MW, Libby P. Increased expression of matrix metalloproteinases and matrix degrading activity in vulnerable regions of human atherosclerotic plaque. Journal of Clinical Investigation 1994;94(6):2493-503.
[173] Wald NJ, Watt HC, Hackshaw AK. Integrated screening for Down's syndrome based on tests performed during the first and second trimesters. New England Journal of Medicine 1999;341(7):461-7.
[174] Cosin-Sales J, Christiansen M, Kaminski P, Oxvig C, Overgaard MT, Cole D, et al. Pregnancy-associated plasma protein A and its endogenous inhibitor, the proform of eosinophil major basic protein (proMBP), are related to complex stenosis morphology in patients with stable angina pectoris. Circulation 2004;109(14):1724-8.
[175] Laterza OF, Cameron SJ, Chappell D, Sokoll LJ, Green GB. Evaluation of pregnancy-associated plasma protein A as a prognostic indicator in acute coronary syndrome patients. Clinica Chimica Acta 2004;348:163-9.
[176] McCann CJ, Glover BM, Menown IBA, Moore MJ, McEneny J, Owens CG, et al. Novel biomarkers in early diagnosis of acute myocardial infarction compared with cardiac troponin T. European Heart Journal 2008;29(23):2843-50.
[177] Dominguez-Rodriguez A, Abreu-Gonzalez P, Garcia-Gonzalez M, Ferrer J, Vargas M. Circulating pregnancy-associated plasma protein A is not an early marker of acute myocardial infarction. Clinical Biochemistry 2005;38:180-2.
[178] Elesber AA, Lerman A, Denktas AE, Resch ZT, Jared Bunch T, Schwartz RS, et al. Pregnancy associated plasma protein-A and risk stratification of patients presenting with chest pain in the emergency department. International Journal of Cardiology 2007;117(3):365-9.
[179] Heeschen C, Dimmeler S, Hamm CW, Fichtlschere S, Simoons ML, Zeiher AM, et al. Pregnancy-associated plasma protein-A levels in patients with acute coronary syndromes: comparison with markers of systemic inflammation, platelet activation, and myocardial necrosis. Journal of the American College of Cardiology 2005;45(2):229-37.
[180] Lund J, Qin QP, Ilva T, Pettersson K, Voipio-Pulkki LM, Porela P, et al. Circulating pregnancy-associated plasma protein A predicts outcome in patients with acute coronary syndrome but no troponin I elevation. Circulation 2003;108(1924):1926.
[181] Sanchis J, Bosch X, Bodi V, Bellera N, Nunez J, Benito B, et al. Combination of clinical risk profile, early exercise testing and circulating biomarkers for evaluation of patients with acute chest pain without ST-segment deviation or troponin elevation. Heart 2008;94(3):311-5.
[182] Sadosty AT, Goyal DG, Boie ET, Chiu CK. Emergency Department D-dimer testing. Journal of Emergency Medicine 2001;21(4):423-9.
[183] Fancher TL, White RH, Kravitz RL. Combined use of rapid D-dimer testing and estimation of clinical probability in the diagnosis of deep vein thrombosis: systematic review. British Medical Journal 2004;329:821-9.

[184] Ridker PM, Hennekens CH, Cerskus A, Stampfer MJ. Plasma concentration of cross-linked fibrin degradation product (D-dimer) and the risk of future myocardial infarction among apparently healthy men. Circulation 1994;90(5):2236-40.
[185] Danesh J, Whincup P, Walker M, Lennon L, Thomson A, Appleby P, et al. Fibrin D-dimer and coroanry heart disease: Prospective study and meta-analysis. Circulation 2001;103:2323-7.
[186] Itakura H, Sobel BE, Boothroyd D, Leung LL, Iribarren C, Go AS, et al. Do plasma biomarkers of coagulation and fibrinolysis differ between patients who have experienced an acute myocardial infarction versus stable exertional angina? American Heart Journal 2007;154(6):1059-64.
[187] Shitrit AB, Tzivony D, Shilon Y, Rudensky B, Sulkes J, Gutterer N, et al. The role of enzyme-linked immunosorbent assay D-dimer in patients with acute coronary syndrome presenting with normal cardiac enzymes. Blood Coagulation & Fibrinolysis 2006;17(8):621-4.
[188] Shitrit D, Shitrit AB, Rudensky B, Sulkes J, Gutterer N, Zviony D. Role of ELISA D-dimer test in patients with unstable angina pectoris presenting at the Emergency Department with a normal electrocardiogram. American Journal of Haematology 2004;77(2):147-50.
[189] Shitrit D, Shitrit AB, Rudensky B, Sulkes J, Tzviony D. Determinants of ELISA D-dimer sensitivity for unstable angina pectoris as defined by coronary catheterization. American Journal of Haematology 2004;76:121-5.
[190] Fiotti N, Di Chiara A, Altamura N, Miccio M, Fioretti P, Guarnieri G, et al. Coagulation indicator in chronic stable effort angina and unstable angina: relationship with acute phase reactants and clinical outcome. Blood Coagulation & Fibrinolysis 2002;13(3):247-55.
[191] Kruskal JB, Commerford PJ, Franks JJ, Kirsch RE. Fibrin and fibrinogen-related antigens in patients with stable and unstable coronary artery disease. The New England Journal of Medicine 1987;317(22):1361-5.
[192] Watanabe R, Wada H, Sakakura M, Mori Y, Nakasaki T, Okugawa Y, et al. Plasma levels of activated protein C-protein C inhibitor complex in patients with hypercoagulable states. American Journal of Haematology 2000;65:35-40.
[193] Kamikura Y, Wada H, Yamada A, Shimura M, Hiyoyama K, Shiku H, et al. Increased tissue factor pathway inhibitor in patients with acute myocardial infarction. American Journal of Haematology 1997;55:183-7.
[194] Oldgren J, Linder R, Grip L, Siegbahn A, Wallentin L. Coagulation Activity and Clinical Outcome in Unstable Coronary Artery Disease. Arteriosclerosis, Thrombosis, and Vascular Biology 2001;21(6):1059-64.
[195] Tello-Montoliu A, Marin F, Roldan V, Mainar L, Lopez MT, Sogorb F, et al. A multimarker risk stratification approach to non-ST elevation acute coronary syndrome: implications of troponin T, CRP, NT pro-BNP and fibrin D-dimer levels. Journal of Internal Medicine 2007;262(6):651-8.
[196] Bayes-Genis A, Mateo J, Santalo M, Oliver A, Guindo J, Badimon L, et al. D-dimer is an early diagnostic marker of coronary ischemia in patients with chest pain. American Heart Journal 2000;140:379-84.

[197] Derhaschnig U, Laggner AN, Roggla M, Hirschl MM, Kapiotis S, Marsik C, et al. Evaluation of coagulation markers for early diagnosis of acute coronary syndromes in the Emergency Room. Clinical Chemistry 2002;48(11):1924-30.
[198] Noal MR, Vargas LCR, Halla J, Da Rocha Silla LM. Lack of association between cardiac troponin T and D-dimer in the evaluation of myocardial damage. Journal of Clinical Laboratory Analysis 2005;19(6):282-4.
[199] Lippi G, Filippozzi L, Montagnana M, Salvagno GL, Guidi GC. Diagnostic value of D-dimer measurement in patients referred to the emergency department with suspected myocardial ischemia. Journal of Thrombosis & Thrombolysis 2008;25(3):247-50.
[200] Hall C. Essential biochemistry and physiology of (NT-pro) BNP. European Journal of Heart Failure 2004;6:257-60.
[201] Maisel AS, Krishnaswamy P, Nowak RM, McCord J, Hollander JE, Duc P, et al. Rapid measurement of B-type natriuretic peptide in the emergency diagnosis of heart failure. New England Journal of Medicine 2002;347:161-7.
[202] Morrison LK, Harrison A, Krishnaswamy P, Kazanegra R, Clopton P, Maisel A. Utility of a rapid B-natriuretic peptide assay in differentiating congestive heart failure from lung disease in patients presenting with dyspnea. Journal of the American College of Cardiology 2002;39(2):202-9.
[203] Omland T, Aakvaag A, Bonarjee WS, Caidahl K, Lie RT, Nilsen DWT, et al. Plasma brain natriuretic peptide as an indicator of left ventricular systolic function and long-term survival after acute myocardial infarction. Circulation 1996;93:1963-9.
[204] Ruck A, Gustaffson T, Norrborn J, Nowak J, Kallner G, Soderberg M, et al. ANP and BNP but not VEGF are regionally overexpressed in ischemic human myocardium. Biochemical and Biophysical Research Communications 2004;322:287-91.
[205] Goetze JP, Gore A, Moller CH, Steinbruchel DA, Rehfeld JF, Nielsen LB. Acute myocardial hypoxia increases BNP gene expression. FASEB Journal 2004;18(15):1928-30.
[206] Marumoto K, Hamada M, Hiwada K. Increased secretion of atrial and brain natriuretic peptides during acute myocardial ischaemia induced by dynamic exercise in patients with angina pectoris. Clinical Science 1995;88:551-6.
[207] Staub D, Nusbaumer C, Zellweger MJ, Jonas N, Wild D, Pfisterer ME, et al. Use of B-type natriuretic peptide in the detection of myocardial ischemia. American Heart Journal 2006;151(6):1223-30.
[208] Sinclair H, Paterson M, Walker S, Beckett G, Fox KA. Predicting outcome in patients with acute coronary syndrome: evaluation of B-type natriuretic peptide and the global registry of acute coronary events (GRACE) risk score. Scottish Medical Journal 2007;52(3):8-13.
[209] Mega JL, Morrow DA, de Lemos JA, Sabatine SA, Rifai N, Gibson CM, et al. B-type natriuretic peptide at presentation and prognosis in patients with ST-segment elevation myocardial infarction. Journal of the American College of Cardiology 2004;44(2):335-9.
[210] de Lemos JA, Morrow DA, Bentley JH, Omland T, Sabatine MS, McCabe CH, et al. The prognostic value of B-type natriuretic peptide in patients with acute coronary syndromes. New England Journal of Medicine 2001;345:1014-21.

[211] Morrow DA, de Lemos JA, Sabatine MS, Murphy A, Demopoulous LA, Di Battiste PM, et al. Evaluation of B-type natriuretic peptide for risk assessment in unstable angina/non-ST-elevation myocardial infarction. B-type natriuretic peptide and prognosis in TACTICS-TIMI. Journal of the American College of Cardiology 2003;41(8):1264-72.
[212] Grabowski M, Filipiak KJ, Malek LA, Karpinski G, Huczek Z, Stolarz P, et al. Admission B-type natriuretic peptide assessment improves early risk stratification by Killip classes and TIMI risk score in patients with acute ST elevation myocardial infarction treated with primary angioplasty. International Journal of Cardiology 2007;115(3):386-90.
[213] Ahmed W, Zafar S, Alam AY, Ahktar N, Shah MA, Alpert MA. Plasma levels of B-type natriuretic Peptide in patients with unstable angina pectoris or acute myocardial infarction: prognostic significance and therapeutic implications. Angiology 2007;58(3):269-74.
[214] Sun T, Wang L, Zhang Y. Prognostic Value of B-type Natriuretic Peptide in Patients with Acute Coronary Syndromes. Archives of Medical Research 2006;37(4):502-5.
[215] Kuklinska AM, Sobkowicz B, Kaminski KA, Mroczko B, Musial WJ, Szmitkowski M, et al. The benefits of repeated measurements of B-type natriuretic peptide in patients with first ST-elevation myocardial infarction treated with primary percutaneous coronary intervention. International Heart Journal 2006;47(6):843-54.
[216] Kuklinska AM, Sobkowicz B, Mroczko B, Sawicki R, Musial WJ, Knapp M, et al. Prognostic significance of the admission plasma B-type natriuretic peptide measurement in patients with first ST-elevation myocardial infarction in comparison with C-reactive protein and TIMI risk score. Clinica Chimica Acta 2007;382(1-2):106-11.
[217] Ketch TR, Turner SJ, Sacrinty MT, Lingle KC, Applegate RJ, Kutcher MA, et al. Derived fibrinogen compared with C-reactive protein and brain natriuretic peptide for predicting events after myocardial infarction and coronary stenting. American Heart Journal 2008;156(2):234-40.
[218] Palazzuoli A, Deckers J, Calabro A, Campagna MS, Nuti R, Pastorelli M, et al. Brain natriuretic peptide and other risk markers for outcome assessment in patients with non-ST-elevation coronary syndromes and preserved systolic function. American Journal of Cardiology 2006;98(10):1322-8.
[219] Gunes Y, Okcun B, Kavlak E, Erbas C, Karcier S. Value of brain natriuretic peptide after acute myocardial infarction. Anadolu Kardiyoloji Dergisi 2008;8(3):182-7.
[220] Mukoyama M, Nakao K, Obata K, Jougasaki M, Yoshimura M, Morita E, et al. Augmented secretion of brain natriuretic peptide in acute myocardial infarction. Biochemical and Biophysical Research Communications 1991;180(1):431-6.
[221] Morita E, Hirofumi Y, Michihiro Y, Ogawa H, Jougasaki M, Matsumura T, et al. Myocardial injury/infarction: increased plasma levels of brian natriuretic peptide in patients with acute myocardial infarction. Circulation 1991;88(1):82-91.
[222] Horio T, Shimada KE, Hokno M, Yoshimura T, Kawabayashi T, Yasunari K, et al. Serial changes in atrial and brain natriuretic peptides in patients with acute myocardial infarction treated with early coronary angioplasty. American Heart Journal 1993;126:293-9.

[223] Kikuta K, Yasue H, Yoshimura M, Morita E, Sumida H, Kato H, et al. Increased plasma levels of B-type natriuretic peptide in patients with unstable angina. American Heart Journal 1996;132:101-7.
[224] Palazzuoli A, Rizzello V, Calabro A, Gallotta M, Martini G, Quatrini I, et al. Osteoprotegerin and B-type natriuretic peptide in non-ST elevation acute coronary syndromes: relation to coronary artery narrowing and plaques number. Clinica Chimica Acta 2008;391(1-2):74-9.
[225] Paelinck BP, Vrints CJ, Bax JJ, Bosmans JM, De Hert SG, de RA, et al. Relation of B-type natriuretic peptide early after acute myocardial infarction to left ventricular diastolic function and extent of myocardial damage determined by magnetic resonance imaging. American Journal of Cardiology 2006;97(8):1146-50.
[226] Brown A, George J, Murphy MJ, Struthers A. Could BNP screening of acute chest pain cases lead to safe earlier discharge of patients with non-cardiac causes? A pilot study. QJM 2007;100(12):755-61.
[227] Bassan R, Potsch A, Maisel A, Tura B, Villacorta H, Nogueira MV, et al. B-type natriuretic peptide: a novel early blood marker of acute myocardial infarction in patients with chest pain and no ST-segment elevation. European Heart Journal 2005;26:234-40.
[228] Hamilton AJ, Swales LA, Neill J, Murphy JC, Darragh KM, Rocke LG, et al. Risk stratification of chest pain patients in the emergency department by a nurse utilizing a point of care protocol. European Journal of Emergency Medicine 2008;15:9-15.
[229] Kwan G, Isakson SR, Beede J, Clopton P, Maisel AS, Fitzgerald RL. Short-term serial sampling of natriuretic peptides in patients presenting with chest pain. Journal of the American College of Cardiology 2007;49(11):1186-92.
[230] Brown AM, Sease KL, Robey JL, Shofer FS, Hollander JE. The impact of B-type natriuretic peptide in addition to troponin I, creatine kinase-MB, and myoglobin on the risk stratification of emergency department chest pain patients with potential acute coronary syndrome. Annals of Emergency Medicine 2007;49(2):153-63.
[231] Glatz JFC, van der Voort D, Hermens WT. Fatty acid-binding protein as the earliest available plasma marker of acute myocardial injury. Journal of Clinical Ligand Assay 2002;25(2):167-77.
[232] Glatz JFC, van Bilsen M, Paulussen RJA, Veerkamp JH, van der Vusse GJ, Reneman RS. Release of fatty acid-binding protein from isolated rat heart subjected to ischemia and reperfusion or to the calcium paradox. Biochimica et Biophysica Acta (BBA) - Lipids and Lipid Metabolism 1988;961(1):148-52.
[233] Tanaka T, Hirota Y, Sohmiya K, Nishimura S, Kawamura K. Serum and urinary human heart fatty acid-binding protein in acute myocardial infarction. Clinical Biochemistry 1991;24(2):195-201.
[234] Mad P, Domanovits H, Fazelnia C, Stiassny K, Russmuller G, Cseh A, et al. Human heart-type fatty-acid-binding protein as a point-of-care test in the early diagnosis of acute myocardial infarction. QJM 2007;100(4):203-10.
[235] Alhashemi JA. Diagnostic accuracy of a bedside qualitative immunochromatographic test for acute myocardial infarction. American Journal of Emergency Medicine 2006;24(2):149-55.

[236] Seino Y, Ogata K, Takano T, Ishii J, Hishida H, Morita H, et al. Use of a whole blood rapid panel test for heart-type fatty acid-binding protein in patients with acute chest pain: comparison with rapid troponin T and myoglobin tests.[see comment]. American Journal of Medicine 115(3):185-90, 2003 Aug 15.

[237] Ghani F, Wu AH, Graff L, Petry C, Armstrong G, Prigent F, et al. Role of heart-type fatty acid-binding protein in early detection of acute myocardial infarction. Clinical Chemistry 2000;46(5):718-9.

[238] Valle HA, Riesgo LGC, Bel MS, Gonazalo FE, Sanchez MS, Oliva LI. Clinical assessment of heart-type fatty acid-binding protein in early diagnosis of acute coronary syndrome. European Journal of Emergency Medicine 2008;15(3):140-4.

[239] Panju AA, Hemmelgam BR, Guyatt GH, Simei DL. The rational clinical examination: Is this patient having a myocardial infarction. JAMA 1998;280(14):1256-63.

[240] Body R, McDowell G, Carley S, Wibberley C, Gerguson J, Mackway-Jones K. A FABP-ulous rule out strategy? Heart fatty acid binding protein and troponin for rapid exclusion of acute myocardial infarction. Resuscitation 2011; 82: 1041-6.

[241] Body R, Carley S, McDowell G, Jaffe AS, France M, Cruickshant K, Wibberley C, Nuttall M, Mackway-Jones K. Rapid exclusion of acute myocardial infarction in patients with undetectable troponin using a high sensitivity assay. J Am Coll Cardiol 2011; 58: 1333-9.

3

Roles of Serotonin in Atherothrombosis and Related Diseases

Takuya Watanabe[1] and Shinji Koba[2]
[1]*Laboratory of Cardiovascular Medicine, Tokyo University of Pharmacy and Life Sciences, Tokyo,*
[2]*Department of Medicine, Division of Cardiology, Showa University School of Medicine, Tokyo, Japan*

1. Introduction

Serotonin (5-hydroxytryptamine, 5-HT) was first identified as a powerful vasoconstrictor over a century ago (Rapport et al., 1948), and in the past 20 years has been recognized as an arterial smooth muscle mitogen (Nemecek et al., 1986). Serotonin is also known to act as a monoaminergic neurotransmitter in the brain and gastrointestinal tract, and is involved in a variety of functions, such as mood regulation, urine storage and voiding, the regulation of sleep and body temperature, food intake, and intestinal motility (Ni & Watts, 2006). Serotonin is predominantly synthesized and secreted into the blood stream by enterochromaffin cells in the gastrointestinal tract and is rapidly taken up and stored in small dense granules in platelets (Fanburg & Lee, 1997). In humans, 90% of the body's 5-HT is located in the intestines, and the rest is present primarily in platelets (8–9%) and the central nervous system (1–2%) (Fanburg & Lee, 1997). When platelets adhere and aggregate at sites of vessel injury, 5-HT is secreted and directly accelerates platelet aggregation (De Clerck, 1990; Wester et al., 1992).

The first step in the synthesis of 5-HT from tryptophan is the enzyme tryptophan hydroxylase (TPH), which is also the rate-limiting enzyme in its biosynthesis. TPH is known to have two isoforms, TPH-1 and TPH-2, which share an overall identity of approximately 70% (Walther et al., 2003). TPH-1 is mainly present in the pineal gland, thymus, spleen, and enterochromaffin cells of the gastrointestinal tract. TPH-2 is expressed solely in neuronal cells, such as the raphe nuclei of the brainstem. Finally, 5-HT is metabolized by monoamine oxidase A to form the metabolite 5-hydroxyindole acetic acid. Monoamine oxidase A is an intracellular enzyme and 5-HT must first be taken up into the cell prior to metabolism, and this achieved via the 5-HT transporter (Ni & Watts, 2006).

Serotonin is an extracellular mediator recognized by the 5-HT transporter and seven different receptors (5-HT_1–5-HT_7), giving rise to pleiotropic intracellular responses. All 5-HT receptors, with the exception of 5-HT_6, are involved in cardiovascular regulation. Central 5-HT_{1A}, 5-HT_3, and 5-HT_7 receptors play physiological roles in the regulation of cardiovascular reflexes, controlling changes in parasympathetic drive to the heart (Ramage

& Villalon, 2008). These reflexes also affect the activity of the sympathetic nervous system, which itself can be inhibited by stimulation of central 5-HT_{1A} receptors causing a drop in blood pressure and excited by 5-HT_2 receptor stimulation resulting in an increase in blood pressure. Acute vascular constriction by 5-HT is usually mediated by 5-HT_{1B} and 5-HT_{2A} receptors, except in the intracranial arteries in which constriction is mediated only through 5-HT_{1B} receptors (Kaumann & Levy, 2006). Both 5-HT_{1B} and 5-HT_{2A} receptors can mediate coronary artery spasm and pulmonary hypertension.

Serotonin promotes platelet aggregation and the proliferation, migration, and contraction of vascular smooth muscle cells (VSMCs). In addition to physiological hemostasis, these vascular responses play pivotal roles in the development and progression of atherothrombotic diseases.

2. Platelet aggregation

When platelets aggregate, 5-HT is released into the extracellular environment from the dense granules of activated platelets. The 5-HT thus released further activates other platelets by binding to 5-HT_{2A} receptors on the platelet membrane, contributing to thrombus formation (Satoh et al., 2006). Serotonin promotes further platelet recruitment and activates the coagulation pathway. The blood vessels in which platelets aggregate are exposed to high concentrations of 5-HT (Benedict et al., 1986).

3. Vasoconstriction

Serotonin is well known to act as a potent vasoconstrictor and has been shown to cause both vasoconstriction and vasodilation by interacting with receptors expressed on VSMCs, endothelial cells, or adrenergic nerve endings. In systemic arterial smooth muscle, 5-HT induces contractions only at sites of endothelial damage where platelet aggregation occurs, and this effect is antagonized by 5-HT_2 receptor antagonists (Sigal et al., 1991). Serotonin also amplifies the effects of other vasoconstrictors, such as histamine, angiotensin II, prostaglandin $F_{2\alpha}$, and noradrenaline (O'Rourke et al., 2006). The potent contractile effect of 5-HT may contribute to the vasoconstriction of coronary collateral vessels developed by reduction of coronary blood flow (Wright et al., 1992) and vasospastic disorders in arteries covered with regenerated endothelium and in atherosclerotic arteries (Sobey et al., 1991). The blood vessel wall chronically exposed to abnormally high blood pressure is characterized by increased vascular responsiveness to 5-HT. Chronic blockade of 5-HT_{2A} receptors reduces the development of hypertension in spontaneously hypertensive rats (Gradin et al., 1991).

4. VSMC proliferation

Serotonin stimulates the migration and proliferation of VSMCs through 5-HT_{2A} receptors (Tamura et al., 1997; Pakala et al., 1997, 1999a). Serotonin interacts synergistically with atherogenic lipoproteins (low-density lipoprotein [LDL] and β-very low density lipoprotein) (Koba et al., 1999, 2000), oxidized LDL and its major components, such as lysophosphatidylcholine, 4-hydroxy-2-nonenal, and reactive oxygen species (Watanabe et al., 2001a, 2001b) in inducing VSMC proliferation. Serotonin also potentiates the mitogenic effects of other vasoactive agents, such as endothelin-1, angiotensin II, urotensin II, and thromboxane A_2 (Watanabe et al., 2001c, 2001d, 2001e; Pakala et al. 1997), platelet-derived microparticles (Pakala, 2004), coagulation factors, such as thrombin and coagulation factor Xa (Pakala & Benedict, 1999; Pakala, 2003), and monocyte chemoattractant protein-1 on VSMCs (Watanabe et al., 2001f). In addition, 5-HT stimulates the expression of interleukin-6 and cyclooxygenase-2 in VSMCs (Ito et al., 2000; Machida et al., 2011).

5. Endothelial cell function

Serotonin stimulates the expression of tissue factor and plasminogen activator inhibitor-1 in endothelial cells through 5-HT_{2A} receptors (Kawano et al., 2001). Serotonin-stimulated endothelial cells secrete a T lymphocyte-specific chemotactic cytokine with competence growth factor activity (Katz et al., 1994). Serotonin, alone and combined with thromboxane A_2, potently induces endothelial cell proliferation (Pakala et al., 1994, 1999b). However, there is still controversy regarding the effects of 5-HT on endothelial cell proliferation (Ruiz-Perez et al., 2011).

6. Macrophage foam cell formation

Serotonin stimulates monocyte adhesion (Lorenowicz et al., 2006), and enhances macrophage foam cell formation associated with increased uptake of oxidized LDL (Aviram et al., 1992) and up-regulation of acyl-coenzyme A:cholesterol acyltransferase-1 (ACAT-1) through 5-HT_{2A} receptors (Suguro et al., 2006).

7. 5-HT_{2A} receptor blockade

The roles of 5-HT in the pathogenesis of atherothrombotic diseases are revealed by the results of pharmacological interventions involving 5-HT_{2A} receptors. Functional analyses of the roles of 5-HT in the cardiovascular system using 5-HT_{2A} receptor knockout mice have not been performed. Several studies performed before the discovery of specific and/or selective 5-HT_{2A} receptor antagonists indicated that 5-HT_2 receptor blockers inhibit angioplasty-induced vasospasm and microvascular constriction following atherosclerotic plaque rupture in atherosclerotic rabbit models (Sigal et al., 1991; Taylor et al., 2004).

Sarpogrelate, a selective 5-HT_{2A} receptor antagonist, inhibits responses to 5-HT mediated by 5-HT_{2A} receptors, such as platelet aggregation and thrombus formation (H Hara et al., 1991a; Nishihira et al., 2006), and prevents the development of atherosclerotic lesions (H Hara et al., 1991b; Hayashi et al., 2003), vasospasm (Miyata et al., 2000), and intimal hyperplasia in vein grafts after bypass grafting (Kodama et al., 2009). This drug suppresses ACAT-1 expression in macrophages (Suguro et al., 2006), vascular oxidative stress and VSMC proliferation (Watanabae et al., 2001d; Sun et al., 2011), up-regulates endothelial nitric oxide synthase (Hayashi et al., 2003), and reduces the expression of matrix metalloproteinase-1 that degrades the arterial extracellular matrix (Hayashi et al., 2003), contributing to stabilization of vulnerable plaque.

8. 5-HT concentration and Cardiovascular Disease

In a previous study involving the measurement of washed platelet-bound 5-HT concentration in three groups based on the presence and absence of thrombotic diseases, platelet 5-HT levels were highest in patients with deep-vein thrombosis and pulmonary embolism prior to death from thrombotic events. The lowest levels were detected in subjects without thrombosis, and intermediate levels were seen in patients with cerebral thrombosis (Misra et al., 1975). These findings suggested that 5-HT plays an important role in the initiation of thrombus formation.

With regard to the association between 5-HT and coronary artery disease (CAD), it has been reported that coronary sinus plasma samples from CAD patients evoked vasoconstriction, whereas systemic artery and venous samples from patients without CAD did not (Rubanyi et al., 1987). In addition, the vasoactive activity of the coronary sinus plasma showed a positive correlation with the severity and extent of coronary artery narrowing, and among various pharmacological interventions only methiothepin, a non-selective 5-HT receptor antagonist, prevented the vasoconstriction induced by these coronary sinus plasma samples. Although this study did not measure 5-HT concentration directly, these results suggested that the amount of 5-HT released into the coronary sinus plays an important role in vasoconstriction in the coronary circulation. The first direct measurement of 5-HT concentration in human coronary circulation was reported by van den Berg and co-workers (van den Berg et al., 1989), who measured 5-HT concentration by modified radioenzymatic assay (Benedict et al., 1986; Hussain & Sole, 1981) in platelet-poor plasma obtained from the central aorta and coronary sinus of 52 patients referred for cardiac catheterization. The 5-HT concentration in the coronary circulation determined by subtracting the levels in the aorta from those in the coronary sinus is significantly higher in patients with CAD compared with those without CAD (0.6 ± 6.6 ng/ml vs. -5.6 ± 10.3 ng/ml, mean ± SD, $p < 0.05$). These concentrations were significantly higher in CAD patients with complex coronary lesions compared with those with smooth concentric lesions (3.1 ± 5.5 ng/ml vs. -1.9 ± 6.6 ng/ml, $p < 0.02$). A similar method was used to measure 5-HT concentration in coronary circulation in 8 patients with CAD undergoing plain old balloon angioplasty (POBA) (Golino et al., 1994). The 5-HT levels in the coronary sinus increased significantly after POBA, while those in the aorta did not change. Coronary constriction distal to the site of dilation observed after POBA was positively correlated with the 5-HT concentration in the coronary circulation, and this coronary constriction was inhibited by pretreatment with the 5-HT_{2A} receptor antagonist, ketanserin. Other studies using similar techniques have shown that the transcardiac 5-HT concentration is significantly higher in patients with variant angina pectoris compared with non-CAD controls (Murakami et al., 1996, 1998). These studies demonstrated that 5-HT released from activated platelets plays an important role in the pathogenesis of CAD in humans. However, the methods used in these studies required invasive procedures.

Vikenes and co-workers measured 5-HT concentrations in platelet rich plasma from venous blood using high-performance liquid chromatography (HPLC) in 122 men undergoing coronary angiography (Vikenes et al., 1999). Their data indicated that total 5-HT concentration was positively correlated with platelet count ($r = 0.552$, $p < 0.001$), and both total 5-HT concentration and platelet counts were significantly higher in patients with CAD compared with those without CAD. The difference in 5-HT level was greatest in men aged ≤ 60 years old, and the difference reduced steadily with age. The high 5-HT concentration ≥ 1 μmol/l was significantly associated with CAD, with an odds ratio (OR) of 3.84 (95% confidence interval [CI] 1.12–13.11), independently of age and smoking. During a mean follow-up period of 44 ± 15 months, Kaplan-Meier cardiac event-free survival curves for

CAD patients aged ≤ 70 years old indicated a better prognosis with regard to cardiac events for patients with low 5-HT (< 1 μmol/l) (log rank test, $p < 0.05$). Venous plasma 5-HT concentration measured by radioimmunoassay was reported to be significantly higher in patients with variant angina pectoris than in those with healed myocardial infarction or controls (Figueras et al., 2005). On the other hand, comparison of 5-HT concentration in platelet-poor plasma and whole blood indicated that plasma 5-HT concentration tended to increase with age, while its concentration in whole blood decreased (K Hara et al., 2004). The ratio of plasma to whole-blood concentration of 5-HT was significantly higher in various types of CAD, such as variant angina pectoris, acute coronary syndrome (ACS), and prior myocardial infarction, compared with healthy controls, whereas whole-blood 5-HT levels were somewhat higher in healthy controls than in patients with effort angina. The ratio of plasma to whole-blood concentration of 5-HT was recently demonstrated to be positively correlated with Framingham 10-year risk scores for CAD (Y Hirowatari et al., 2011). These clinical studies suggested that high levels of 5-HT are significantly associated with atherosclerotic cardiovascular diseases and the occurrence of cardiovascular events. Thus, 5-HT plays a key role in the pathogenesis of atherothrombosis.

9. 5-HT$_{2A}$ receptor blocker and treatment of CAD

Several clinical studies with 5-HT$_{2A}$ receptor blockers have supported the experimental results demonstrating that 5-HT plays an important role in the development of CAD due to platelet aggregation, VSMC constriction, and migration and proliferation of VSMCs. In a study of 22 patients with stable effort angina, oral administration of 200 mg of sarpogrelate 1 hour prior to treadmill exercise test was shown to improve exercise capacity and the severity score determined by myocardial perfusion scintigraphy in 12 patients with well-developed collateral flow evaluated by coronary angiography, whereas sarpogrelate affected neither exercise time nor severity score in other patients without collateral flow (Tanaka et al., 1998). This was confirmed in another study involving 2 weeks of treatment with 300 mg of sarpogrelate in 20 patients with stable angina pectoris (Kinugawa et al., 2002); treatment with sarpogrelate significantly increased the specific activity scale score, increased exercise time and rate-pressure product, an index of myocardial oxygen consumption, at onset of ischemic ST depression ≥ 0.1 mV on electrocardiogram, and decreased the number of anginal attacks only in patients with angiographically proven well-developed collateral flow. On the other hand, sarpogrelate showed no effects in the patients without well-developed collateral flow. Similar results were obtained in another study with intravenous injection of another 5-HT$_{2A}$ receptor antagonist, ketanserin (Kyriakides et al., 1999). In a study of stable angina pectoris patients with single-vessel disease, ketanserin increased coronary collateral blood flow and decreased myocardial ischemia during POBA. In a study of 15 CAD patients without significant stenosis (< 75% diameter stenosis) in the left anterior descending coronary artery, oral administration of 200 mg of sarpogrelate increased the coronary blood flow velocity at both baseline and hyperemia evaluated by intracoronary Doppler guidewire without any effects on systemic blood pressure or cardiac output (Satomura et al., 2002). On the other hand, there were no significant differences in baseline or hyperemic coronary blood flow velocity in the control group. These results suggested that sarpogrelate augments coronary flow reserve by inhibiting 5-HT-induced coronary vasoconstriction and platelet aggregation in collateral vessels in CAD patients.

In a comparative study of the effects of oral administration of sarpogrelate administration (200 mg) or placebo in addition to aspirin and ticlopidine 60 minutes before POBA in 20 patients with stable effort angina with a de novo single stenotic lesion of 75%–90%, length < 20 mm in the proximal left anterior descending coronary artery, sarpogrelate significantly reduced the ischemic ST changes after coronary angioplasty compared with the placebo group with no changes in collateral blood flow, blood pressure, or heart rate (Horibe et al., 2004). These observations suggested that sarpogrelate improves myocardial ischemic injury by pharmacological ischemic preconditioning rather than by stimulating collateral development.

Studies investigating the effects of 5-HT_{2A} receptor blockers on prevention of restenosis after coronary angioplasty yielded conflicting results between ketanserin and sarpogrelate. In a small placebo-controlled study, 24-hour infusion of ketanserin following POBA prevented the early restenosis evaluated at 24 hours after POBA but failed to prevent restenosis at 4 to 9 months after POBA (Klein et al., 1990). The Post-Angioplasty Restenosis Ketanserin (PARK) study was a randomized, double-blind, placebo-controlled trial to assess the effects of ketanserin in prevention of restenosis after POBA (Serruys et al., 1993). A total of 658 patients with stable or unstable angina pectoris who were scheduled to undergo elective POBA received either ketanserin (loading dose, 40 mg 1 hour before POBA; maintenance dose, 40 mg bid for 6 months) or placebo. All patients received aspirin for 6 months. The primary clinical end points were defined as any one of the following: cardiac death, myocardial infarction, or the need for repeat angioplasty or bypass surgery of the previously dilated sites between the first POBA and 6 months after POBA. The relative risk of the primary end points for the ketanserin group compared with the placebo group was 0.89 (95% CI 0.70–1.13). The restenosis rate according to > 50% stenosis and the quantitative angiographic findings were similar between the two groups. The PARK study failed to show that ketanserin could prevent restenosis and improve clinical outcome after POBA. On the other hand, in an investigation of the effects of sarpogrelate in prevention of restenosis after coronary stenting in Japanese patients with stable angina pectoris, pretreatment with sarpogrelate for 3 days before coronary stenting and continuation of 300 mg of sarpogrelate for 6 months in addition to 81 mg of aspirin and 200 mg of ticlopidine markedly reduced restenosis rate at 6 months after coronary stenting compared with the non-sarpogrelate treatment group (4.3% vs. 28.6%, $p < 0.005$) (Fujita et al., 2003). The results of multivariate logistic regression analysis showed that treatment with sarpogrelate was a significant predictor for angiographic restenosis, independent of the findings of quantitative coronary angiography, stent characteristics, and the presence of diabetes. These two studies differed in 5-HT_{2A} receptor blocker drug characteristics and pretreatment period as well as the angioplasty procedure. The latter study supported the suggestion that sarpogrelate may prevent the development of intimal hyperplasia due to VSMC proliferation. Further randomized controlled trials to investigate the effects of sarpogrelate on prevention of restenosis after placement of drug-eluting stents are required.

10. 5-HT_{2A} receptor blocker and treatment of Peripheral Artery Disease

Sarpogrelate is widely used clinically as an anti-platelet drug for prevention of thrombosis and treatment of critical limb ischemic symptoms in patients with peripheral artery disease (PAD), such as arteriosclerosis obliterans (ASO) and Buerger's disease. In a study by

Miyazaki and colleagues (Miyazaki et al., 2007), 22 patients with PAD received either sarpogrelate at a dose of 300 mg orally or conventional therapy for 12 weeks. Both forearm and leg endothelium-dependent vasodilation were improved and maintained for 24 weeks in patients treated with sarpogrelate whereas no improvement was observed in patients treated with conventional therapy. In addition, endothelium-nondependent vasodilation was similar between the two treatment groups. These results suggest that 12 weeks of treatment with sarpogrelate improved vascular endothelial function in PAD patients. Further they investigated the effects of a combination of bone marrow mononuclear cell implantation and sarpogrelate on endothelial function in 16 PAD patients (Higashi et al., 2010). They performed the evaluations before and after bone marrow mononuclear cell implantation in 16 patients with critical limb ischemia. A 12-week course of sarpogrelate treatment amplified the increased leg blood flow responses to acetylcholine evaluated by plethysmography induced by bone marrow mononuclear cell implantation compared with conventional treatment, whereas bone marrow mononuclear cell implantation improved limb ischemic symptoms in the sarpogrealate group as well as in the conventional treatment group. These two studies showed that a treatment with sarpogrelate for at least 12 weeks has a beneficial effect on vascular endothelial function in PAD patients treated with conventional therapy.

There have been several small studies of the effects of sarpogrelate on various biomarkers without controls in PAD patients. In a study of 13 patients with ASO, treatment with sarpogrelate for 1 week decreased adenosine diphosphate (ADP)- or collagen-induced platelet aggregation and reduced the releases of platelet-derived growth factor, soluble P-selectin, and transforming growth factor-β1 from platelets stimulated by ADP or collagen (Nakamura et al., 2001). In a study of 24 non-diabetic and non-medicated diabetic patients with PAD (Fontaine grades 1 and 2), 300 mg of sarpogrelate decreased insulin resistance at 2 weeks and 3 months after treatment, and increased plasma levels of adiponectin at 3 months after treatment (Kokubu, 2006). Similarly, 300 mg of sarpogrelate increased adiponectin levels at 2 and 3 months after treatment in 8 diabetic patients with ASO (Yamakawa et al., 2003). Treatment with 300 mg of sarpogrelate improved limb ischemic symptoms and decreased interleukin-18 levels in 8 diabetic patients with ASO (Yamakawa et al., 2004). In a study of 10 patients with Buerger's disease, 8 weeks of treatment with 300 mg of sarpogrelate was well-tolerated. However, platelet aggregation induced by 5-HT increased significantly after 2 and 4 weeks, and whole-blood 5-HT concentration increased significantly after 2 weeks of treatment (Rydzewski et al, 1996).

11. 5-HT_{2A} receptor blocker and treatment of ischemic cerebrovascular disease

There have been no reports of high plasma 5-HT levels in patients with stroke at the acute phase. In a study of elderly subjects, plasma 5-HT concentration measured by enzyme immunoassay was significantly higher in patients with vascular dementia caused by stroke or atherosclerotic small vessel disease compared with age-matched controls (Ban et al., 2007).

In a double-blind, controlled, clinical-pharmacological study, 47 patients with ischemic stroke who discontinued any antiplatelet agents and anticoagulants or fibrinolytic agents, were randomly assigned to receive one of three daily doses of sarpogrelate, i.e., 75, 225, or 300 mg, for 7 days (Uchiyama et al., 2007). Sarpogrelate treatment inhibited platelet aggregation induced by 5-HT plus adrenaline in a dose-dependent manner. The Sarpogrelate-Aspirin Comparative Clinical Study for Efficacy and Safety in Secondary Prevention of Cerebral Infarction (S-ACCESS) trial was a randomized, double-blind, controlled trial to evaluate and compare the efficacy and safety of sarpogrelate with those of aspirin for prevention of recurrence in patients with ischemic stroke (Shinohara et al., 2008). A total of 1050 patients with recent ischemic stroke (1 week to 6 months after onset) were randomly allocated to receive either 300 mg of sarpogrelate or 81 mg of aspirin with a mean duration of follow-up of 1.59 years (maximum: 3.37 years). The annual recurrence rates of cerebral infarction were 6.09% (95% CI 4.83–7.67) with sarpogrelate and 4.86% (3.75–6.28) with aspirin. The hazard ratio (HR) was 1.25 (95% CI 0.89–1.77); the upper limit of 95% CI of the HR exceeded 1.33, indicating that sarpogrelate was slightly inferior to aspirin in preventing the recurrence of cerebral infarction. On the other hand, the incidence rates of serious vascular events, defined as stroke, ACS, or vascular event-related death, were similar between the sarpogrelate and aspirin group. There were significantly fewer bleeding events in the sarpogrelate group compared with the aspirin group (11.9%, 95% CI 9.6–14.4 vs. 17.3%, 14.7–20.2, respectively, $p < 0.005$). In subgroup analysis in the S-ACCESS trial, sarpogrelate was shown to be inferior to aspirin in most subgroups except diabetic patients (Shinohara & Nishimaru, 2009). Thus, sarpogrelate may be a useful treatment option for Japanese stroke patients with diabetes.

12. Conclusion

This review presented a discussion of the potential involvement of 5-HT mediated through 5-HT_{2A} receptors in the development of atherothrombotic cardiovascular diseases, including platelet aggregation, thrombus formation, VSMC contraction, and arterial intimal hyperplasia. These responses are synergistically augmented with other vasoactive compounds, atherogenic lipids, and various inflammatory cytokines. The 5-HT_{2A} receptor antagonists inhibit the 5-HT-mediated atherothrombotic process. Although ketanserin inhibits not only 5-HT_{2A} receptors but also α1-adrenergic and histamine H_1 receptors, it was withdrawn due to its tendency to induce proarrhythmia. Sarpogrelate is a specific 5-HT_{2A} receptor antagonist that has been reported to have various beneficial effects especially in patients with CAD and/or atherosclerotic cardiovascular disease with diabetes, and to have fewer adverse effects compared with other anti-platelet agents. However, larger randomized controlled trials of sarpogrelate in CAD, PAD, stroke, and diabetes are required.

13. Acknowledgments

We thank Dr. Claude R. Benedict and Dr. Rajbabu Pakala for their many insightful comments and kind support in our research.

14. References

Aviram, M.; Fuhrman, B.; Maor, I. & Brook, G.J. (1992). Serotonin increases macrophage uptake of oxidized low density lipoprotein. *Eur J Clin Chem Clin Biochem* 30, pp. 55-61

Ban, Y.; Watanabe, T.; Miyazaki, A.; Nakano, Y.; Tobe, T.; Idei, T.; Iguchi, T.; Ban, Y. & Katagiri T. (2007). Impact of increased plasma serotonin levels and carotid atherosclerosis on vascular dementia. *Atherosclerosis* 195, pp. 153-159

Benedict, C.R.; Mathew, B.; Rex, K.A.; Cartwright, J. & Sordahl, L.A. (1986). Correlation of plasma serotonin changes with platelet aggregation in an in vivo dog model of spontaneous occlusive coronary thrombus formation. *Circ Res* 58, pp. 58-67

De Clerck, F. (1990). The role of serotonin in thrombogenesis. *Clin Physiol Biochem* 8 (Suppl 3), pp. 40-49

Fanburg, B.L. & Lee, S.L. (1997). A new role for an old molecule: serotonin as mitogen. *Am J Physiol* 272, pp. L795-806

Figueras, J.; Domingo, E.; Cortadellas, J.; Padilla, F.; Dorado, D.G.; Segura, R.; Galard, R. & Soler, J.S. (2005). Comparison of plasma serotonin levels in patients with variant angina pectoris versus healed myocardial infarction. *Am J Cardiol* 96, pp. 204-207

Fujita, M.; Mizuno, K.; Ho, M.; Tsukahara, R.; Miyamoto, A.; Miki, O.; Ishii, K. & Miwa, K. (2003). Sarpogrelate treatment reduces restenosis after coronary stenting. *Am J Heart J* 145, pp. E16

Golino, P.; Piscione, F.; Benedict, C.R.; Anderson, H.V.; Cappelli-Bigazzi, M.; Indolfi, C.; Condorelli, M.; Chiariello, M. & Willerson, J.T. (1994). Local effect of serotonin released during coronary angioplasty. *N Engl J Med* 330, pp. 523-528

Gradin, K.; Hedner, T. & Persson, B. (1991). Antihypertensive effects of chronic 5-hydroxytryptamine (5-HT2) receptor blockade with irindalone in the spontaneously hypertensive rat. *J Neural Transm Gen Sect* 83, pp. 227-233

Hara, H.; Kitajima, A.; Shimada, H. & Tamao, Y. (1991a). Antithrombotic effect of MCI-9042, a new antiplatelet agent on experimental thrombosis models. *Thromb Haemost* 66, pp. 484-488

Hara, H.; Shimada, H.; Kitajima, A. & Tamao, Y. (1991b). Effect of (+/-)-2-(dimethylamino)-1-[[o-(m-methoxyphenethyl)phenoxy] methyl]ethyl hydrogen succinate on experimental models of peripheral obstructive disease. *Arzneimittelforschung* 41, pp. 616-620

Hara, K.; Hirowatari, Y.; Yoshika, M.; Komiyama, Y.; Tsuka, Y. & Takahashi, H. (2004). The ratio of plasma to whole-blood serotonin may be a novel marker of atherosclerotic cardiovascular disease. *J Lab Clin Med* 144, pp. 31-37

Hayashi, T.; Sumi, D.; Matsui-Hirai, H.; Fukatsu, A.; Arockia, J.; Rani, P.J.A.; Kano, H.; Tsunekawa, T. & Iguchi, A. (2003). Sarpogrelate HCl, a selective 5-HT_{2A} antagonist, retards the progression of atherosclerosis through a novel mechanism. *Atherosclerosis* 168, pp. 23-31

Higashi, Y.; Miyazaki, M.; Goto, C.; Sanada, H.; Sueda, T. & Chayama, K. (2010). Sarpogrelate hydrochloride, a selective 5-hydroxytryptamine(2A) antagonist, augments autologous bone marrow mononuclear cell implantation-induced improvement in endothelium-dependent vasodilation in patients with critical limb ischemia. *J Cardiovasc Pharmacol* 55, pp. 56-61

Hirowatari, Y.; Hara, K.; Shimura, Y. & Takahashi, H. (2011). Serotonin levels in platelet-poor plasma and whole blood from healthy subjects: relationship with lipid markers and coronary heart disease risk score. *J Atheroscler Thromb* 18, pp. 874-882

Horibe, E.; Nishigaki, K.; Minatoguchi, S. & Fujiwara, H. (2004). Sarpogrelate, a 5-HT_2 receptor blocker, may have a preconditioning-like effect in patients with coronary artery disease. *Circ J* 68, pp. 68-72

Hussain, M.N. & Sole, M.J. (1981). A simple, specific, radioenzymatic assay for picogram quantities of serotonin or acetylserotonin in biological fluids and tissues. *Anal Biochem* 111, pp. 101-110

Ito, T.; Ikeda, U.; Shimpo, M.; Yamamoto, K. & Shimada, K. (2000). Serotonin increases interleukin-6 synthesis in human vascular smooth muscle cells. *Circulation* 102, pp. 2522-2527

Katz, M.F.; Farber, H.W.; Dodds-Stitt, Z.; Cruikshank, W.W. & Beer, D.J. (1994). Serotonin-stimulated aortic endothelial cells secrete a novel T lymphocyte chemotactic and growth factor. *J Leukoc Biol* 55, pp. 567-573

Kaumann, A.J. & Levy, F.O. (2006). 5-hydroxytryptamine receptors in the human cardiovascular system. *Pharmacol Ther* 111, pp. 674-706

Kawano, H.; Tsuji, H.; Nishimura, H.; Kimura, S.; Yano, S.; Ukimura, N.; Kunieda, Y.; Yoshizumi, M.; Sugano, T.; Nakagawa, K.; Masuda, H.; Sawada, S. & Nakagawa, M. (2001). Serotonin induces the expression of tissue factor and plasminogen activator inhibitor-1 in cultured rat aortic endothelial cells. *Blood* 97, pp. 1697-1702

Kinugawa, T.; Fujita, M.; Lee, J.D.; Nakajima, H.; Hanada, H. & Miyamoto, S. (2002). Effectiveness of a novel serotonin blocker, sarpogrelate, for patients with angina pectoris. *Am Heart J* 144, pp. E1

Klein, W.; Eber, B.; Dusleag, J.; Rotman, B.; Költringer, P.; Luha, O. & Vanhoutte, P.M. (1990). Ketanserin prevents early restenosis following percutaneous transluminal coronary angioplasty. *Clin Physiol Biochem* 8 (Suppl 3), pp. 101-107

Koba, S.; Pakala, R.; Watanabe, T.; Katagiri, T. & Benedict, C.R. (1999). Vascular smooth muscle proliferation: synergistic interaction between serotonin and low density lipoproteins. *J Am Coll Cardiol* 34, pp. 1644-1651

Koba, S.; Pakala, R.; Katagiri, T. & Benedict C.R. (2000). Hyperlipemic-very low density lipoprotein, intermediate density lipoprotein and low density lipoprotein act synergistically with serotonin on vascular smooth muscle cell proliferation. *Atherosclerosis* 149, pp. 61-67

Kodama, A.; Komori, K.; Hattori, K.; Yamanouchi, D.; Kajikuri, J. & Itoh, T. (2009). Sarpogrelate hydrochloride reduced intimal hyperplasia in experimental rabbit vein graft. *J Vasc Surg* 49, pp. 1272-1281

Kokubu, N.; Tsuchihashi, K.; Yuda, S.; Hase, M.; Eguchi, M.; Wakabayashi, T.; Hashimoto, A.; Nakata, T.; Miura, T.; Ura, N.; Nagao, K.; Tsuzuki, M.; Wakabayashi, C. & Shimamoto, K. (2006). Persistent insulin-sensitizing effects of sarpogrelate hydrochloride, a serotonin 2A receptor antagonist, in patients with peripheral arterial disease. *Circ J* 70, pp.1451-1456

Kyriakides, Z.S.; Sbarouni, E.; Nikolaou, N.; Antoniadis, A. & Kremastinos, D.T. (1999). Intracoronary ketanserin augments coronary collateral blood flow and decreases myocardial ischemia during balloon angioplasty. *Cardiovasc Drugs Ther* 13, pp. 415-422

Lorenowicz, M.J.; van Gils, J.; de Boer, M.; Hordijk, P.L. & Fernandez-Borja M. (2006). Epac1-Rap1 signaling regulates monocyte adhesion and chemotaxis. *J Leukoc Biol* 80, pp. 1542-1552

Machida, T.; Ohta, M.; Onoguchi, A.; Iizuka, K.; Sakai, M.; Minami, M. & Hirafuji, M. (2011). 5-Hydroxytryptaime induces cyclooxygenase-2 in rat vascular smooth muscle cells: mechanisms involving Src, PKC and MAPK activation. Eur J Pharmacol 656, pp. 19-26

Misra, D.P.; Staddon, G.; Jackson, P.; Powell, N. & Misra, J. (1975). Platelet 5-hydroxy-tryptamine in thrombotic and non-thrombotic diseases. *Age Ageing* 4, pp. 105-109

Miyata, K.; Shimokawa, H.; Higo, T.; Yamawaki, T.; Katsumata, N.; Kandabashi, T.; Tanaka, E.; Takamura, Y.; Yogo, K.; Egashira, K. & Takeshita, A. (2000). Sarpogrelate, a selective 5-HT_{2A} serotonergic receptor antagonist, inhibits serotonin-induced coronary artery spasm in a porcine model. *J Cardiovasc Pharmacol* 35, pp. 294-301

Miyazaki, M.; Higashi, Y.; Goto, C.; Chayama, K.; Yoshizumi, M.; Sanada, H.; Orihashi, K. & Sueda, T. (2007). Sarpogrelate hydrochloride, a selective 5-HT_{2A} antagonist, improves vascular function in patients with peripheral arterial disease. *J Cardiovasc Pharmacol* 49, pp. 221-227

Murakami, Y.; Ishinaga, Y.; Sano, K.; Murakami, R.; Kinoshita, Y.; Kitamura, J.; Kobayashi, K.; Okada, S.; Matsubara, K.; Shimada, T. & Morioka, S. (1996). Increased serotonin release across the coronary bed during a nonischemic interval in patients with vasospastic angina. *Clin Cardiol* 19, pp. 473-476

Murakami, Y.; Shimada, T.; Ishinaga, Y.; Kinoshita, Y.; Kin, H.; Kitamura, J.; Ishibashi, Y. & Murakami, R. (1998). Transcardiac 5-hydroxytryptamine release and impaired coronary endothelial function in patients with vasospastic angina. *Clin Exp Pharmacol Physiol* 25, pp. 999-1003

Nakamura, K.; Kariyazono, H.; Masuda, H.; Sakata, R. & Yamada, K. (2001). Effects of sarpogrelate hydrochloride on adenosine diphosphate- or collagen-induced platelet responses in arteriosclerosis obliterans. *Blood Coagul Fibrinolysis* 12, pp. 391-397

Nemecek, G.M.; Coughlin, S.R.; Handley, D.A. & Moskowitz, M.D. (1986). Stimulation of aortic smooth muscle cell mitogenesis by serotonin. *Proc Natl Acad Sci USA* 83, pp. 674-678

Ni, W. & Watts, S.W. (2006). 5-Hydroxytryptamine in the cardiovascular system: focus on the serotonin transporter (SERT). *Clin Exp Pharmacol Physiol* 33, pp. 575-583

Nishihira, K.; Yamashita, A.; Tanaka, N.; Kawamoto, R.; Imamura, T.; Yamamoto, R.; Eto, T. & Asada, Y. (2006). Inhibition of 5-hydroxytryptamine2A receptor prevents occlusive thrombus formation on neointima of the rabbit femoral artery. *J Thromb Haemost* 4, pp. 247-255

O'Rourke, S.T.; Vanhoutte, P.M. & Miller, V.M. (2006). Vascular pharmacology, In: *Vascular Medicine: a Companion to Braunwald's Heart Disease*, Creger, M.A.; Dzau, V.J.; Loscalzo, J. pp. 71-100, Saunders Elsevier, Philadelphia, Pennsylvania, USA

Pakala, R.; Willerson, J.T. & Benedict, C.R. (1994). Mitogenic effect of serotonin on vascular endothelial cells. *Circulation* 90, pp. 1919-1926

Pakala, R.; Willerson, J.T. & Benedict, C.R. (1997). Effect of serotonin, thromboxane A_2, and specific receptor antagonists on vascular smooth muscle cell proliferation. *Circulation* 96, pp. 2280-2286

Pakala, R. & Benedict, C.R. (1999). Synergy between thrombin and serotonin in inducing vascular smooth muscle cell proliferation. *J Lab Clin Med* 134, pp. 659-667

Pakala, R.; Pakala, R.; Sheng W.L. & Benedict, C.R. (1999a). Eicosapentaenoic acid and docosahexaenoic acid block serotonin-induced smooth muscle cell proliferation. *Arterioscler Thromb Vasc Biol* 19, pp. 2316-2322

Pakala, R.; Pakala, R.; Sheng W.L. & Benedict, C.R. (1999b). Serotonin fails to induce proliferation of endothelial cells preloaded with eicosapentaenoic acid and docosahexaenoic acid. *Atherosclerosis* 145, pp. 137-146

Pakala, R. (2003). Coagulation factor Xa synergistically interacts with serotonin in inducing vascular smooth muscle cell proliferation. *Cardiovasc Radiat Med* 4, pp. 69-76

Pakala, R. (2004). Serotonin and thromboxane A_2 stimulate platelet-derived microparticle-induced smooth muscle cell proliferation. *Cardiovasc Radiat Med* 5, pp. 20-26

Ramage, A.G. & Villalon, C.M. (2008). 5-hydroxytryptamine and cardiovascular regulation. *Trends Pharmacol Sci* 29, pp. 472-481

Rapport, M.M.; Green, A.A. & Page, I.H. (1948). Serum vasoconstrictor (serotonin). IV. Isolation and characterization. *J Biol Chem* 176, pp. 1243-1251

Rubanyi, G.M.; Frye, R.L.; Holmes, D.R. Jr. & Vanhoutte, P.M. (1987). Vasoconstrictor activity of coronary sinus plasma from patients with coronary artery disease. *J Am Coll Cardiol* 9, pp. 1243-1249

Ruiz-Perez, M.V.; Sanchez-Jimenez, F.; Quesada, A.R. & Medina, M.A. (2011). A re-evaluation of the mitogenic effect of serotonin on vascular smooth muscle cells. *J Biol Regul Homeost Agents* 25, pp. 13-20

Rydzewski, A.; Urano, T.; Hachiya, T.; Kaneko, H.; Baba, S.; Takada, Y. & Takada, A. (1996). The effect of a $5HT_2$ receptor antagonist sarpogrelate (MCI-9042) treatment on platelet function in Buerger's disease. *Thromb Res* 84, pp. 445-452

Satoh, K.; Yatomi, Y. & Ozaki, Y. (2006). A new method for assessment of an anti-$5HT_{2A}$ agent, sarpogrelate hydrochloride, on platelet aggregation. *J Thromb Haemost* 4, pp. 479-481

Satomura, K.; Takase, B.; Hamabe, A.; Ashida, K.; Hosaka, H.; Ohsuzu, F. & Kurita, A. (2002). Sarpogrelate, a specific 5-HT2-receptor antagonist, improves the coronary microcirculation in coronary artery disease. *Clin Cardiol* 25, pp. 28-32

Serruys, P.W.; Klein, W.; Tijssen, J.P.; Rutsch, W.; Heyndrickx, G.R.; Emanuelsson, H.; Ball, S.G.; Decoster, O.; Schroeder, E.; Liberman, H.; Eichhorn, E.; Willerson, J.T.; Anderson, H.V.; Khaja, F.; Alexander, R.W.; Baim, D.; Melkert, R.; van Oene, J.C. & Van Gool, R. (1993). Evaluation of ketanserin in the prevention of restenosis after percutaneous transluminal coronary angioplasty. A multicenter randomized double-blind placebo-controlled trial. *Circulation* 88, pp. 1588-1601

Shinohara, Y.; Nishimaru, K.; Sawada, T.; Terashi, A.; Handa, S.; Hirai, S.; Hayashi, K.; Tohgi, H.; Fukuuchi, Y.; Uchiyama, S.; Yamaguchi, T.; Kobayashi, S.; Kondo, K.; Otomo, E. & Gotoh, F.; S-ACCESS Study Group. (2008). Sarpogrelate-Aspirin Comparative Clinical Study for Efficacy and Safety in Secondary Prevention of Cerebral Infarction (S-ACCESS): A randomized, double-blind, aspirin-controlled trial. *Stroke* 39, pp.1827-1833

Shinohara, Y. & Nishimaru, K.; S-ACCESS study group. (2009). Sarpogrelate versus aspirin in secondary prevention of cerebral infarction: differential efficacy in diabetes? Subgroup analysis from S-ACCESS. *Stroke* 40, pp. 2862-2865

Sigal, S.L.; Gellman, J.; Sarembock, I.J.; LaVeau, P.J.; Chen, Q.; Cabin, H.S. & Ezekowitz, M.D. (1991). Effects of serotonin-receptor blockade on angioplasty-induced vasospasm in an atherosclerotic rabbit model. *Arterioscler Thromb* 11, pp. 770-783

Sobey, C.G.; Dusting, G.J. & Woodman, O.L. (1991). Enhaced vasoconstriction by serotonin in rabbit carotid arteries with atheroma-like lesions in vivo. *Clin Exp Pharmacol Physiol* 18, pp. 367-370

Suguro, T.; Watanabe, T.; Kanome, T.; Kodate, S.; Hirano, T.; Miyazaki, A. & Adachi, M. (2006). Serotonin acts as an up-regulator of acyl-coenzyme A:cholesterol acyltransferase-1 in human monocyte-macrophages. *Atherosclerosis* 186, pp. 275-281

Sun, Y.M.; Su, Y.; Jin, H.B.; Li, J. & Bi, S. (2011). Sarpogrelate protects against high glucose-induced endothelial dysfunction and oxidative stress. *Int J Cardiol* 147, pp. 383-387

Tamura, K.; Kanzaki, T.; Saito, Y.; Otabe, M.; Saito, Y. & Morisaki, N. (1997). Serotonin (5-hydroxytryptamine, 5-HT) enhances migration of rat aortic smooth muscle cell through 5-HT_2 receptors. *Atherosclerosis* 132, pp. 139-143

Tanaka, T.; Fujita, M.; Nakae, I.; Tamaki, S.; Hasegawa, K.; Kihara, Y.; Nohara, R. & Sasayama S. (1998). Improvement of exercise capacity by sarpogrelate as a result of augmented collateral circulation in patients with effort angina. *J Am Coll Cardiol* 32, pp. 1982-1986

Taylor, A.J.; Bobik, A.; Berndt, M.C.; Kannelakis, P. & Jennings G. (2004). Serotonin blockade protects against early microvascular constriction following atherosclerotic plaque rupture. *Eur J Pharmacol* 486, pp. 85-89

Uchiyama, S.; Ozaki, Y.; Satoh, K.; Kondo, K. & Nishimaru, K. (2007). Effect of sarpogrelate, a 5-HT(2A) antagonist, on platelet aggregation in patients with ischemic stroke: clinical-pharmacological dose-response study. *Cerebrovasc Dis* 24, pp. 264-70

Van den Berg, E.K.; Schmitz, J.M.; Benedict, C.R.; Malloy, C.R.; Willerson, J.T. & Dehmer, G.J. (1989). Transcardiac serotonin concentration is increased in selected patients with limiting angina and complex coronary lesion morphology. *Circulation* 79, pp. 116-124

Vikenes, K.; Farstad, M. & Nordrehaug, J.E. (1999). Serotonin is associated with coronary artery disease and cardiac events. *Circulation* 100, pp. 483-489

Walther, D.J.; Peter, J.U.; Bashammakh, S.; Hörtnagl, H.; Voits, M.; Fink, H. & Bader, M. (2003). Synthesis of serotonin by a second tryptophan hydroxylase isoform. *Science* 299, pp. 76

Watanabe, T.; Pakala, R.; Koba, S.; Katagiri, T. & Benedict, C.R. (2001a). Lysophosphatidylcholine and reactive oxygen species mediate the synergistic effect of mildly oxidized LDL with serotonin on vascular smooth muscle cell proliferation. *Circulation* 103, pp. 1440-1445

Watanabe, T.; Pakala, R.; Katagiri, T. & Benedict, C.R. (2001b). Lipid peroxidation product 4-hydroxy-2-nonenal acts synergistically with serotonin in inducing vascular smooth muscle cell proliferation. *Atherosclerosis* 155, pp. 37-44

Watanabe, T.; Pakala, R.; Katagiri, T. & Benedict, C.R. (2001c). Angiotensin II and serotonin potentiate endothelin-1-induced vascular smooth muscle cell proliferation. *J Hypertens* 19, pp. 731-739

Watanabe, T.; Pakala, R.; Katagiri, T. & Benedict, C.R. (2001d). Serotonin potentiates angiotensin II-induced vascular smooth muscle cell proliferation. *Atherosclerosis* 159, pp. 269-279

Watanabe, T.; Pakala, R.; Katagiri, T. & Benedict, CR. (2001e). Synergistic effect of urotensin II with serotonin on vascular smooth muscle cell proliferation. *J Hypertens* 19, pp. 2191-2196

Watanabe, T.; Pakala, R.; Katagiri, T. & Benedict, C.R. (2001f). Monocyte chemotactic protein 1 amplifies serotonin-induced vascular smooth muscle cell proliferation. *J Vasc Res* 38, pp. 341-349

Wester, P.; Dietrich, W.D.; Prado, R.; Watson, B.D. & Globus, M.Y.T. (1992). Serotonin release into plasma during common carotid artery thrombosis in rats. *Stroke* 23, pp. 870-875

Wright L.; Homans, D.C.; Laxson, D.D.; Dai, X.Z. & Bache, R.J. (1992). Effect of serotonin and thromboxane A2 on blood flow through moderately well developed coronary collateral vessels. *J Am Coll Cardiol* 19, pp.687-693

Yamakawa, J.; Takahashi, T.; Itoh, T.; Kusaka, K.; Kawaura, K.; Wang, X.Q. & Kanda, T. (2003). A novel serotonin blocker, sarpogrelate, increases circulating adiponectin levels in diabetic patients with arteriosclerosis obliterans. *Diabetes Care* 26, pp. 2477-2478

Yamakawa, J.; Takahashi, T.; Saegusa, S.; Moriya, J.; Itoh, T.; Kusaka, K.; Kawaura, K.; Wang, X.Q. & Kanda, T. (2004). Effect of the serotonin blocker sarpogrelate on circulating interleukin-18 levels in patients with diabetes and arteriosclerosis obliterans. *J Int Med Res* 32, pp. 166-169

4

Endothelial Progenitor Cell in Cardiovascular Diseases

Po-Hsun Huang
Division of Cardiology, Taipei Veterans General Hospital, Cardiovascular Research Center, National Yang-Ming University, Taipei, Taiwan

1. Introduction

The last decade has seen a huge interest in the field of regenerative biology, with particular emphasis on the use of isolated or purified stem and progenitor cells to restore structure and function to damaged organs. Circulating endothelial progenitor cells (EPCs) have been studied as a potential cell source that contributes to neovascularization via postnatal vasculogenesis (Asahara et al., 1997). EPCs are reported to naturally home and integrate into sites of physiological vessel formation *in vivo* and incorporate into the vasculature of tumors, ischemic skeletal and cardiac muscle (Asahara et al., 1999). Furthermore, Accumulating evidence demonstrates a relationship between the frequency of circulating EPCs and cardiovascular disease risk (Hill et al., 2003). In the following, we will review the putative role of EPCs in endothelial repair and provides evidence for their influence on atherosclerosis.

2. Identification of EPCs

Despite the availability of effective preventive measures, coronary artery disease (CAD) remains a leading cause of morbidity and mortality in most industrialized countries. Convincing evidence indicates that the integrity and functional activity of the endothelial monolayer play an important role in atherogenesis. Traditional view suggests that endothelium integrity is maintained by neighboring mature endothelial cells which migrate and proliferate to restore injured endothelial cells. However, a series of clinical and basic studies prompted by the discovery of bone marrow-derived EPCs have provided new insights into these processes and demonstrate that the injured endothelial monolayer is regenerated partly by circulating EPCs. Putative circulating endothelial progenitors were first described in the adult human by Asahara *et al.* (Asahara et al., 1997) in 1997. They used the presence of CD34 to sort cells from the adult peripheral blood mononuclear component, based on the knowledge that this antigen is carried by both the angioblasts and haemopoietic stem cells responsible for vasculogenesis in embryonic life. By culturing MNCs (mononuclear cells) enriched or depleted in these $CD34^+$ cells, they showed that the $CD34^+$ component is able to give rise to spindle-shaped cells after 3 days, which become attached to fibronectin. Such culture led to an up-regulation of endothelial lineage markers such as CD31, Flk-1 and Tie2, and loss of the pan-leucocyte CD45 antigen, in these attaching cells. Asahara *et al.* (Asahara et al., 1999) went on to deliver labelled, CD34$^+$-enriched, MNCs into mouse and rabbit models of hindlimb ischemia and demonstrated neovascularization in the relevant limb with apparent incorporation of labelled cells into capillary walls. In separate experiments, they delivered murine labelled-MNCs enriched for Flk-1 and similarly found incorporation into capillaries and small arteries in the mouse hindlimb ischemia model. Carriage of CD31 and lectin binding was observed in these incorporated cells. These landmark studies suggest that circulating EPCs in adult peripheral blood could differentiate into cells of endothelial lineage and enhance revascularization through vasculogenesis.

3. Issues of definition for EPCs

Since these important findings, an enormous amount of research has been undertaken into EPCs; however, in attempting to collate and interpret these results, a major limiting factor is that no simple definition of EPCs exists at the present time, and various methods to define EPC have been reported. This pertains to the unresolved issue of how EPCs should best be defined.

3.1 Antigen-based definitions of EPC

The first method of classification of EPC is based on expression of cell-surface antigens, typically using flow cytometry to quantify relevant populations. Endothelial cells (EC) display a characteristic combination of such antigens, including CD34, KDR (kinase insert domain-containing receptor, a type of VEGFR2), VE-cadherin, vWF (von Willebrand factor) and E-selectin. In order to distinguish mature endothelial cells from circulating endothelial progenitors, some groups have additionally used other antigens which are lost during maturation of endothelial lineage cells, most commonly CD133 (also termed AC133) (Hristov & Weber, 2004). The combination of CD34, KDR and CD133 has been used by several investigators, although many others have used only two of these three. Unfortunately, even with use of all three, this phenotype is not entirely specific, since this same cluster of antigens may also be found on haemopoietic stem cells (Adams & Scadden, 2006; Verfaillie, 2002). This relates to the probable origin of haemopoietic and EC lines from a common precursor, termed the haemangioblast. As haemopoietic stem cells differentiate, CD34, KDR and CD133 antigens are down-regulated and disappear. Furthermore, the use of CD133 to make the distinction from mature ECs will also lead to the exclusion of 'more mature' EPCs which may have lost this marker, while not yet being terminally differentiated. To complicate matters further, while the use of antigenic combinations may have logical appeal, whether this approach actually identifies a group of precursors capable of producing ECs has recently been challenged (Case et al., 2007).

3.2 Culture-based definitions of EPC

The second commonly employed definition for EPCs derives from *in vitro* culture work. Asahara *et al.* described *in vitro* culture of CD34-enriched MNCs leading to the formation of spindle-shaped attaching cells within 3 days (Asahara et al., 1997). Co-culture of CD34-enriched and CD34-depleted cells gave rise, within 12 hours, to multiple clusters, containing round cells centrally and sprouts of spindle-shaped cells at the periphery. This cluster appearance was reminiscent of the blood islands previously described, wherein angioblasts surround hematopoeitic stem cells as the initial stage of vasculogenesis (Flamme & Risau,

1992). Various culture preparations have been used to encourage endothelial lineage proliferation from human blood-derived MNCs. There has been a considerable variation in the details of techniques used: for example, some have replated the adherent cells after 2 days initial culture, whereas others have used the non-adherent cells at this time (Vasa, 2001). Then, endothelial cell lineage was confirmed by indirect immunostaining with the use of DiI-acLDL and co-staining with BS-1 lectin. However, controversy exists with respect to the identification and the origin of EPCs, which are isolated from peripheral blood mononuclear cells by cultivation in medium favoring endothelial differentiation.

4. Early and Late outgrowth EPCs

EPCs can be isolated, cultured, and differentiated ex vivo from the circulating mononuclear cells (MNCs) and exhibit characteristic endothelial properties and markers. Currently, two types of EPCs, namely early and late outgrowth EPCs, can be derived and identified from peripheral blood. The early EPCs appear after 3-5 days of culture, are spindle-shaped, have peak growth at approximately 2 weeks and die by 4 weeks. These have been variously termed 'early EPCs' by Gulati et al. (Gulati et al., 2003) and Hur et al. (Hur et al., 2004), 'attaching cells' by Asahara et al. (Asahara et al., 1997) and CACs (circulating angiogenic cells) by Rehman et al. (Rehman et al., 2003). The second type of EPCs appears only after longer culture, of approximately 2-3 weeks, forming a cobblestone monolayer with near-complete confluence, and can show exponential population growth without senescence over 4-8 weeks and live for up to 12 weeks. These were termed 'late EPCs' by Hur *et al.* (Hur et al., 2004) or OECs by Lin *et al.* (Lin et al., 2000) and Gulati *et al.* (Gulati et al., 2003). Early and late outgrowth EPCs (OECs) share some endothelial phenotype similarities but show different morphology, proliferation rate, survival features, and functions in neovascularization. For clarity, we will use the terms early EPCs and OECs in the present review.

Early EPCs, in contrast, do not participate in tube-forming assays, have only weak invasive ability on gels and produce only low levels of NO. They do, however, demonstrate some features in keeping with an endothelial lineage such as acetylated LDL uptake and lectin binding. In addition, early EPCs do not develop into OECs upon prolonged culture. Among antigenic markers, CD14 (a monocytic marker) has been found by several groups on early EPCs (Romagnani et al., 2005; Urbich et al., 2003). Early EPCs lack the impressive replicative ability of OECs, but are prolific producers of several growth factors, cytokines and chemokines, including VEGF, HGF (hepatocyte growth factor), G-CSF (granulocyte colony-stimulating factor) and GM-CSF (granulocyte/macrophage colony-stimulating factor). The lineage origin of these two culture-derived endothelial-type cells has been examined. Expression of the pan-leucocyte antigen CD45 is relatively greatest in MNCs, lower in early EPCs and lowest in OECs. It appears that early EPCs are mostly derived from a $CD14^+$ population of MNCs, implying a monocytic, rather than true endothelial, lineage (Yoon et al., 2005). In contrast, OECs derive exclusively, or almost exclusively, from the $CD14^-$ population of MNCs (Yoon et al., 2005). It has been suggested that the MNCs from which OECs are derived may represent a 'true' circulating endothelial precursor (angioblasts).

OECs have many similarities to mature ECs, in terms of surface antigens (including KDR, vWF, and VE-cadherin) and high levels of NO (nitric oxide) production by eNOS (endothelial NO synthase). They are able to participate effectively in tube-forming assays *in vitro*. However, OECs differ from mature ECs in having far greater proliferative ability *in vitro* and greater angiogenic potential *in vivo*. A small population of OECs with the highest proliferative potential was able to produce more than 200 progeny per replated cell. Based on these findings, these features make OECs attractive candidates for therapeutic use in ischemia-related neovascularization.

5. Endothelial progenitor cells and atherosclerosis

The discovery of endothelial progenitors within adult peripheral blood presents another possible means of vascular maintenance, namely a reservoir of circulating cells which can home to sites of injury and restore endothelial integrity thus allowing continued normal function. Hill *et al.* (Hill et al., 2003) studied men without known cardiovascular disease but with varying degrees of estimated cardiovascular risk. Endothelial function was determined by using brachial artery flow-mediated vasodilation, and EPC numbers were measured using their CFU assay in study subjects. An inverse correlation was found between numbers of CFUs and the overall Framingham risk score of the participants. Furthermore, they found a positive correlation between the number of EPCs and endothelial function as assessed by brachial artery reactivity of the subjects. These findings are compatible with the hypothesis that an adequate pool of EPCs in the blood may be a key requirement for appropriate endothelial function. It appears that bone marrow-derived EPCs play a pivotal role in the maintenance of adult vascular endothelium. However, the basis of this correlation between EPC levels and endothelial function remains to be determined.

Although the critical role of circulating EPCs in the pathogenesis of atherosclerotic diseases is substantiated by several observations, the relationship between circulating EPCs and coronary artery disease (CAD) remains a subject of debate. Several studies have examined the association between circulating EPCs and CAD or risk factors predisposing to coronary artery disease. Vasa *et al.* reported that the circulating EPCs levels were significantly reduced in patients with CAD compared to those without CAD (Vasa et al., 2001). Wang and coworkers indicated that decreased number and activity of EPCs were observed in patients with stable CAD, and EPC levels were negatively correlated with the severity of coronary stenosis assessed by Gensini score (Wang et al., 2007). Fadini *et al.* also reported that EPCs were significantly reduced in subjects with increased intima-media thickness (Fadini et al., 2006), implying that depletion of EPCs may be an independent predictor of subclinical atherosclerosis. However, Guven *et al.* showed that increased EPCs levels were associated with the presence of significant CAD, and EPC numbers correlated with maximum angiographic stenosis severity (Guven et al., 2006). The apparent conflicting results between different studies may have many explanations, including fundamental differences in the methodologies used to identify circulating EPCs in different studies; heterogeneity of patient population, and effect of the disease stage on biological properties of circulating EPC levels. Based on the angiographic classifications by Syntax score, our recent work has shown that severe CAD patients (with higher Syntax Score) have decreased circulating EPCs numbers than mild CAD patients and subjects with normal angiographic results (unpublished data). Moreover, circulating EPC levels were shown to be negatively correlated with the SXscore in patients with angiographic evidence of CAD. These findings are consistent with a recent study showing that lower level of circulating EPCs predicts CAD progression (Briguori et al., 2010), suggesting the critical role of EPCs in the pathogenesis of CAD.

6. Anti-atherosclerotic actions of EPC

Rapid and complete restoration of endothelial integrity and function prevents development and growth of a neointimal lesion; however, inadequate response to injury will instead allow the formation of an atheromatous lesion. The discovery of circulating endothelial progenitors has led to the theory that they are important mediators of this repair arm, and hence that a depletion or dysfunction in these cells would result in an imbalance between endothelial injury and repair, favoring atherosclerosis. Schmidt-Lucke *et al.* (Schmidt-Lucke et al., 2005) followed up a group of 120 individuals, comprising normal subjects and also patients with either stable or unstable coronary artery disease. They found that major cardiovascular events, CABG (coronary artery bypass grafting) or ischemic stroke were significantly more frequent in the subgroup with lower levels of circulating CD34/KDR double-positive cells at baseline. This association persisted after accounting for conventional cardiovascular risk factors. Werner *et al.* (Werner et al., 2005) studied CD34/KDR double-positive cell numbers in a cohort of 519 patients diagnosed with coronary artery disease by angiography. After adjustment for confounding variables, higher levels of EPCs were associated with a reduced risk of death from cardiovascular causes and of occurrence of a first cardiovascular event at 12 months follow-up. The authors followed up the outcomes when patients were grouped by baseline levels of CFUs (i.e. a culture-based definition of colony formation). Higher CFU formation was associated with a reduced occurrence of a first major cardiovascular event and reduced revascularization at follow-up. However, as discussed above, recent work on the CFU assay suggests that it is assessing the *in vitro* activity of cells which may be relevant to vascular function, but which are not actually EPCs themselves (Rohde et al., 2007; Hur et al., 2007).

Moreover, there is relevant animal-based work in this area of progenitor cells and endothelial function. Wassmann *et al.* (Wassmann et al., 2006) studied endothelial function in ApoE-knockout mice, on a high-cholesterol diet, with atherosclerotic plaques and demonstrable endothelial dysfunction of aortic rings *ex vivo*. They showed that the intravenous administration of spleen-derived MNCs improved endothelium-dependent vasodilation. In addition, Gulati *et al.* (Gulati et al., 2003). used a rabbit model of balloon injury to the carotid arteries. They cultured peripheral blood MNCs in endothelial growth medium for 2 weeks, producing endothelial-phenotype cells carrying CD31 and eNOS, and delivered these culture-modified cells immediately after balloon injury. They found that, compared with saline-treated controls, local treatment with EPCs led to accelerated re-endothelialization and improved endothelial function. Whether the improvement in endothelial function is directly due to increased numbers of new ECs or an indirect effect on pre-existing cells or a papacrine effect by implantation of EPCs remains unclear; however, an increase in vascular NOS activity was documented and is likely to mediate the effect.

7. Therapeutic implications and perspective

A crucial target in the treatment or prevention of atherosclerosis is to promote and maintain the integrity and health of endothelium. Since EPCs play a role in maintaining an intact and functional endothelium, decreased and dysfunctional EPCs may contribute to endothelial dysfunction and susceptibility to atherosclerosis. Enhancement of the regenerative capacity of the injured endothelium seems one way to reduce the incidence of atherosclerotic lesions (Hristov & Weber, 2007). Transplantation of human cord blood-derived EPCs was reported to contribute to neovascularization in various ischemic diseases, and EPC transplantation on diabetic wounds has a beneficial effect, mainly achieved by their direct paracrine action on keratinocytes, fibroblasts, and endothelial cells, rather than through their physical engraftment into host tissues (vasculogenesis). In the TOPCARE-AMI (i.e., "Transplantation of Progenitor Cells and Regeneration Enhancement in Acute Myocardial Infarction") trial (Assmus et al., 2002), intracoronary infusion of cultured human EPCs in patients with recent myocardial infarction was associated with improvements in global left ventricular function and microvascular function. In addition, an EPC-conditioned medium was shown to be therapeutically equivalent to EPCs, at least for the treatment of diabetic dermal wounds (Kim et al., 2010).

There are several ways to increase levels of circulating EPCs and improve their function by pharmacological strategies and lifestyle modification. Notably, it was shown that the angiotensin-converting enzyme (ACE) inhibitors such as ramipril (Min et al., 2004), and angiotensin II (AT II) inhibitors, like valsartan (Bahlmann et al., 2005) increased EPC levels in patients, probably interfering with the CD26/dipeptidylpeptidase IV system. Our recent data showed that moderate intake of red wine significantly enhanced circulating EPC levels and improved EPC functions by modifying NO bioavailability (Huang et al., 2010). Other studies indicated that either the phosphatidylinositol 3-kinase/Akt/endothelial nitric oxide synthase/NO (*PI3K/Akt/eNOS/NO*) signaling pathway or the interaction between hyperglycemia and hyperlipidemia in diabetic patients who have vascular diseases, are potential therapeutic targets for abolishing the impaired function of EPCs (Wang et al., 2011). Neutralization of the $p66^{ShcA}$gene, which regulates the apoptotic response to oxidative stress, prevented high glucose-induced EPC impairment *in vitro* (Di et al., 2009). The existence of molecules acting on EPCs can be used to positively condition cultured EPCs before therapeutic transplantation. Thus, because it is known that chemokine SDF-1α is able to mobilize EPCs, and because EPCs are known to have receptors for SDF-1α, it was demonstrated that SDF-1α - primed EPCs exhibit increased adhesion to HUVEC, resulting in more efficient incorporation of EPCs into sites of neovascularization (Zemani et al., 2008).

8. Conclusions

In conclusion, EPCs are biomarkers of endothelial repair with therapeutic potential, since low EPC levels predict endothelial dysfunction and a poor clinical outcome. Various studies have focused on the important role of EPCs in vasculogenesis and angiogenesis of ischemic tissue in peripheral artery disease as well as acute myocardial infarction, but only a few studies have concentrated on the role of EPCs in the prevention and therapy of atherosclerosis.

9. Acknowledgements

This study was supported in part by research grants from the UST-UCSD International Center of Excellence in Advanced Bio-engineering NSC-99-2911-I-009-101 from the National Science Council; VGH-V98B1-003 and VGH-V100E2-002 from Taipei Veterans General Hospital, and also a grant from the Ministry of Education "Aim for the Top University" Plan.

10. References

Adams, G. & Scadden, D. (2006). The hematopoietic stem cell in its place. *Nat Immunol,* Vol.7; No.4, pp. 333-337,

Asahara, T., et al., (1997). Isolation of putative progenitor endothelial cells for angiogenesis. *Science,* Vol.275, No.5302, pp. 964-967,

Asahara, T., et al., (1999). Bone marrow origin of endothelial progenitor cells responsible for postnatal vasculogenesis in physiological and pathological neovascularization. *Circ Res,* Vol.85; No.3, pp. 221-228,

Assmus, B., et al. (2002). Transplantation of Progenitor Cells and Regeneration Enhancement in Acute Myocardial Infarction (TOPCARE-AMI). *Circulation.* Vol.106; No.24, pp. 3009-3017,

Bahlmann, F., et al. (2005). Stimulation of endothelial progenitor cells: a new putative therapeutic effect of angiotensin II receptor antagonists. *Hypertension.* Vol. 45; No.4, pp. 526-529,

Briguori, C., et al. (2010). Correlations between progression of coronary artery disease and circulating endothelial progenitor cells. *FASEB J.* Vol.24; No.6, pp. 1981-1988,

Case, J., et al. (2007). Human $CD34^+AC133^+VEGFR\text{-}2^+$ cells are not endothelial progenitor cells but distinct, primitive hematopoietic progenitors. *Exp Hematol,* Vol.35; No.7, pp. 1109-1118,

Di, S., et al. (2009). p66ShcA modulates oxidative stress and survival of endothelial progenitor cells in response to high glucose. *Cardiovasc Res.* Vol.82; No.3, pp. 421-429,

Fadini, G., et al. (2006). Peripheral blood cd34+kdr+ endothelial progenitor cells are determinants of subclinical atherosclerosis in a middle-aged general population. *Stroke.* Vol.37, No.9, pp. 2277-2282,

Flamme, I. & Risau, W. (1992). Induction of vasculogenesis and hematopoiesis in vitro. Development, Vol.116; No.2, pp. 435-439,

Gulati, R., et al. (2003). Diverse origin and function of cells with endothelial phenotype obtained from adult human blood. *Circ Res.* Vol.93; No.11, pp. 1023-1025,

Gulati, R., et al. (2003). Autologous culture-modified mononuclear cells confer vascular protection after arterial injury. Circulation. Vol.108; No.12, pp. 1520-1526,

Guven, H., et al. (2006). The number of endothelial progenitor cell colonies in the blood is increased in patients with angiographically significant coronary artery disease. *J Am Coll Cardiol.* Vol.48, No.8, pp. 1579-1587,

Hill, J., et al., (2003). Circulating Endothelial Progenitor Cells, Vascular Function, and Cardiovascular Risk. *N Engl J Med,* Vol.348; No.7, pp. 593-600,

Hristov, M. & Weber, C. (2004). Endothelial progenitor cells: characterization, pathophysiology, and possible clinical relevance. *J Cell Mol Med,* Vol.8; No.4, pp. 498-508,

Hristov, M. & Weber, C. (2007). Endothelial progenitor cells: Cellular biomarkers in vascular disease. *Disease Mechanisms.* Vol.5, pp. 267-271,

Huang, P., et al. (2010). Intake of red wine increases the number and functional capacity of circulating endothelial progenitor cells by enhancing nitric oxide bioavailability. Arterioscler Thromb Vasc Biol. Vol.30; No.4, pp. 869-877,

Hur, J., et al. (2004). Characterization of two types of endothelial progenitor cells and their different contributions to neovasculogenesis. *Arterioscler Thromb Vasc Biol.* Vol.24; No.2, pp. 288-293,

Hur, J., et al. (2007). Identification of a novel role of T cells in postnatal vasculogenesis: characterization of endothelial progenitor cell colonies. *Circulation.* Vol.116; No.15, pp. 1671-1682,

Kim, J., et al. (2010). Human cord blood-derived endothelial progenitor cells and their conditioned media exhibit therapeutic equivalence for diabetic wound healing. *Cell Transplant.* Vol.19, No.12, pp. 1635-1644,

Lin, Y., et al. (2000). Origins of circulating endothelial cells and endothelial outgrowth from blood. *J Clin Invest.* Vol.105; No.1, pp. 71-77,

Min, T., et al. (2004). Improvement in endothelial progenitor cells from peripheral blood by ramipril therapy in patients with stable coronary artery disease. *Cardiovasc Drugs Ther.* Vol.18, No.3, pp. 203-209,

Rehman, J., et al. (2003). Peripheral blood 'endothelial progenitor cells' are derived from monocyte/macrophages and secrete angiogenic growth factors. *Circulation.* Vol.107; No.8, pp. 1164-1169,

Rohde, E., et al. (2007). Immune cells mimic the morphology of endothelial progenitor colonies in vitro. *Stem Cells.* Vol.25; No.7, pp. 1746-1752,

Romagnani, P., et al. (2005). $CD14^{+}CD34$-low cells with stem cell phenotypic and functional features are the major source of circulating endothelial progenitors. *Circ Res.* Vol.97; No.4, pp. 314-322,

Schmidt-Lucke, C., et al. (2005). Reduced number of circulating endothelial progenitor cells predicts future cardiovascular events: proof of concept for the clinical importance of endogenous vascular repair. *Circulation.* Vol.111; No.22, pp. 2981-2987,

Urbich, C., et al. (2003). Relevance of monocytic features for neovascularization capacity of circulating endothelial progenitor cells. *Circulation.* Vol.108; No.20, pp. 2511-2516,

Vasa, M., et al. (2001). Number and migratory activity of circulating endothelial progenitor cells inversely correlate with risk factors for coronary artery disease. *Circ Res.* Vol.89; No.1, pp. 1-7,

Verfaillie, C. (2002). Hematopoietic stem cells for transplantation. *Nat Immunol,* Vol.3; No.4, pp. 314-317,

Wang, H., et al. (2007). Circulating endothelial progenitor cells, c-reactive protein and severity of coronary stenosis in chinese patients with coronary artery disease. *Hypertens Res.* Vol.30, No.2, pp. 133-141,

Wang, R., et al. (2011). Activation of vascular BK channels by docosahexaenoic acid is dependent on cytochrome P450 epoxygenase activity. *Cardiovasc Res.* Vol.90; No.2, pp. 344-352,

Wassmann, S., et al. (2006). Improvement of endothelial function by systemic transfusion of vascular progenitor cells. *Circ Res.* Vol.99; No.8, pp. 74-83,

Werner, N., et al. (2005). Circulating endothelial progenitor cells and cardiovascular outcomes. *N Engl J Med.* Vol.353; No.10, pp. 999-1007,

Yoon, C., et al. (2005). Synergistic neovascularization by mixed transplantation of early endothelial progenitor cells and late outgrowth endothelial cells: the role of angiogenic cytokines and matrix metalloproteinases. *Circulation.* Vol.112, No.11, pp. 1618-1627,

Zemani, F., et al. (2008). Ex vivo priming of endothelial progenitor cells with SDF-1 before transplantation could increase their proangiogenic potential. *Arterioscler Thromb Vasc Biol.* Vol.28; No.4, pp. 644-650,

5

CD40 Ligand and Its Receptors in Atherothrombosis

Daniel Yacoub[1], Ghada S. Hassan[1], Nada Alaadine[1], Yahye Merhi[2] and Walid Mourad[1*]

[1]*Laboratoire d'Immunologie Cellulaire et Moléculaire, Centre Hospitalier de l'Université de Montréal, Hôpital Saint-Luc, Montréal,*

[2]*Institut de Cardiologie de Montréal, Université de Montréal, Montréal, Canada*

1. Introduction

Atherothrombosis is the main underlying determinant of cardiovascular diseases, which remain the leading cause of death in developed countries. Multiple lines of evidence now support the concept of atherothrombosis as a chronic inflammatory disease of the arterial wall.[1, 2] This process involves a complex interplay between modified lipids and cells of the immune and vascular system, which usually evolves into the formation of atherosclerotic lesions yielding a stable necrotic plaque. If left untreated, plaque rupture and thrombosis may ensue, leading to important clinical manifestations, such as acute coronary syndromes and sudden death.[3]

As the incorporation of modified low-density lipoproteins in the arterial wall represents a important step in the onset of atherothrombosis, the subsequent recruitment and activation of inflammatory cells, including monocytes, B- and T-lymphocytes, neutrophils and platelets play a critical role in the pathogenesis of this disease.[4] These cells exhibit pro-atherogenic functions through multiple co-stimulatory and immune molecules present on their cell surface. Among these, the CD40L/CD40 receptor-ligand pair has been the focus of much attention, such that this dyad is now regarded as a pivotal contributor to all underlying phases of atherothrombosis.[5-7] Indeed, the CD40L/CD40 interaction exerts a wide array of biological functions at the forefront of the pathophysiology of this disease and disruption of this cascade by both pharmacological and genetic approaches have shown beneficial results in animal and clinical studies.[8-11] While CD40L is known to mainly interact with its classical receptor CD40, additional binding partners have been described, namely the integrins $\alpha_{IIb}\beta_3$, $\alpha_M\beta_2$ and $\alpha_5\beta_1$. This chapter discusses the role of CD40L and its receptors in the pathophysiology of atherothrombosis, while highlighting its therapeutic potentials in the treatment of this chronic inflammatory disease.

* Corresponding Author

2. The CD40L system

2.1 CD40L

CD40L, also known as CD154, is a 39 kDa transmembrane protein belonging to the tumor necrosis factor (TNF) superfamily originally identified on cells of the immune system.[12, 13] The interaction of CD40L with its respective receptor on B cells, CD40, a glycoprotein also from the TNF receptor (TNFR) family, is of critical importance for immunoglobulin isotype switching during the immune response.[14] The importance of this interaction is highlighted by the pathophysiological manifestations seen in patients suffering from the X-linked hyper-immunoglobulin-M syndrome, in which B-cells fail to produce the immunoglobulin's IgG, IgA and IgE as a consequence of a genetic mutation in the CD40L gene.[15] Because of its wide distribution across cells of the vascular system (endothelium, B and T lymphocytes, neutrophils, platelets, monocytes, dentritic cells and smooth muscle cells), the CD40L/CD40 dyad also shares important implications in cell-mediated immunity. CD40L-induced signaling in these cells leads to the up-regulation of adhesion and co-stimulatory molecules, and the production of pro-inflammatory cytokines, chemokines, growth factors, matrix metalloproteinases (MMPs) and procoagulants.[16-19] These cellular events are also the main mechanisms by which CD40L regulates numerous inflammatory disorders, in particular atherothrombosis and its related complications. In fact, circulating levels of soluble CD40L (sCD40L), which originate from the proteolytic cleavage of membrane-bound CD40L at the surface of activated platelets, have now emerged as strong indicators of cardiovascular events such as atherothrombosis and acute coronary syndromes.[20-22]

2.2 CD40L receptors

CD40

CD40 is the classical high affinity receptor for CD40L. It is constitutively or inducibly expressed by most cells of the vascular system (hematopoietic and non-hematopoietic cells) and represents the main signaling molecule in the CD40L/CD40 receptor-ligand pair.[23] The cytoplasmic domain of CD40 bears signaling domains required for the association of binding proteins termed TNF receptor-associated factors (TRAFs).[24] During humoral immunity, a tight interplay between dendritic cells, T-lymphocytes and B-lymphocytes occurs, throughout which the activation of CD40 provides a crucial signal for the activation, differentiation and secretion of immunoglobulins by B cells.[25] Moreover, CD40 activation in these cells induces an important anti-apoptotic signal that facilitates cell survival and differentiation, primarily through activation of the anti-apoptotic proteins Bcl-XL, A20, Bfl-1 and Mcl-1, which protect against Fas ligand and TNF-induced cell death.[26] As discussed above, CD40 signaling plays a significant role in cell-mediated immunity, an important aspect by which the CD40L/CD40 dyad initiates and exacerbates atherosclerotic lesions. For instance, CD40 activation on endothelial cells induces the up-regulation of a plethora of proinflammatory adhesion molecules, cytokines, chemokines, matrix metalloproteinases and procoagulants.[16] In addition, it has been demonstrated that upon CD40L binding CD40 activation on platelets can enhance platelet function and promote the secretion of inflammatory cytokines involved in plaque formation (this aspect will be discussed in greater detail bellow).[27-29]

CD40-TRAF dependent signaling

The engagement of CD40 by CD40L promotes the clustering of CD40 and induces the association of TRAFs to the cytoplasmic domain of CD40.[30] These adapter proteins are essential for the activation of different signaling pathways including the canonical and non-canonical nuclear factor κB (NF-κB)-signaling pathways and the activation of mitogen-activated protein kinases (MAPKs).[30] The TRAF family comprises six known members, among which TRAF-1, -2, -3, -5 and -6 have been shown to drive CD40-dependent cellular responses.

TRAF-1 can only bind weakly to the cytoplasmic tail of CD40 and therefore regulates the signaling of others TRAF members, in particular TRAF-2.[30, 31] Indeed, TRAF-1 deficiency in antigen presenting cells and B-lymphocytes leads to a significant reduction in the recruitment of TRAF-2 to CD40, indicating that TRAF-1 facilitates the association of TRAF-2 to the cytoplasmic domain of CD40.[32, 33] In agreement with these results, it has been shown that the recruitment of both TRAF-1 and TRAF-2 are required for complete activation of NF-κB in B-cells, since the knockout of both genes results in a greater inhibition of the NF-κB signaling pathway, in comparison to single knockouts.[33]

TRAF-2 is an important contributor to CD40 signaling and its major role resides in the activation of the NF-κB signaling pathway, as well as the activation of the p38, Akt and JNK MAPKs. CD40 bears a direct binding site for TRAF-2 and blockage of this interaction leads to immune deficiencies such as B-cell proliferation and isotype switching.[24, 34] Despite its significant implications in CD40 signaling, TRAF-2 deficiency may be overcome by TRAF-6 activation. This was confirmed by data showing that binding of either TRAF-2 or TRAF-6 alone may activate the NF-κB pathway, while inhibition of both these members completely abolishes CD40-dependant B-cell activation, suggesting that both members collaborate for the activation of this critical signaling cascade.[35-37]

TRAF-3 functions as a negative regulator of CD40 signaling through its constitutive association with TRAF-2.[38, 39] In absence of stimulation, TRAF-3 interacts with TRAF-2, which allows the degradation of the NF-κB inducing kinase (NIK) protein, a critical stimulator of NF-κB.[40] TRAF-3 deficiency in B cells exacerbates NF-κB and JNK activation, primarily through cytosolic accumulation of NIK, thus confirming the negative regulatory functions of TRAF-3 in B cells.[41]

Very little information is available regarding the role of TRAF-5 in CD40 signaling. Nevertheless, it appears that TRAF-5 can interact with TRAF-3 to modulate NF-κB activation in B cells. This was shown by experiments in which TRAF-5 deficiency diminishes NF-κB activation, causing a reduction in cell activation, expression of co-stimulatory molecules and antibody production.[42, 43]

TRAF-6 plays a significant role in the activation of key CD40-dependent signaling pathways, such as NF-κB, p38, JNK and Akt.[44] As discussed above, TRAF-6 synergizes with TRAF-2 in order to regulate the activation of NF-κB. Although TRAF-6 contains a direct binding site for CD40, specific inhibition of this domain shows lesser inhibitory effects than ablation of the complete protein, indicating that TRAF-6 may still have a functional role in CD40 signaling without binding directly to CD40.[30, 45] Indeed, one of the main functions of TRAF-6 resides in its ability to interact with TRAF-2, which is already bound to CD40, and facilitate the activation of downstream targets.

Recently, a study aiming at evaluating the implication of TRAF members in neointima formation, a critical step of atherothrombosis, was conducted. Using a CD40 transgenic mouse model, in which mutations at the TRAF2/3/5, TRAF6 or TRAF2/3/5/6 binding sites were carried out, the authors conclude that the CD40-TRAF6 axis is a key regulator of inflammatory cell infiltration and neointima formation at sites of vascular injury.[46]

Although most vascular complications associated to CD40L, including atherothrombosis, have been largely attributed to its interaction with CD40, recently identified additional receptors merit attention. These include the integrins $\alpha_{IIb}\beta_3$, $\alpha_5\beta_1$ and $\alpha_M\beta_2$ and (Figure 1).

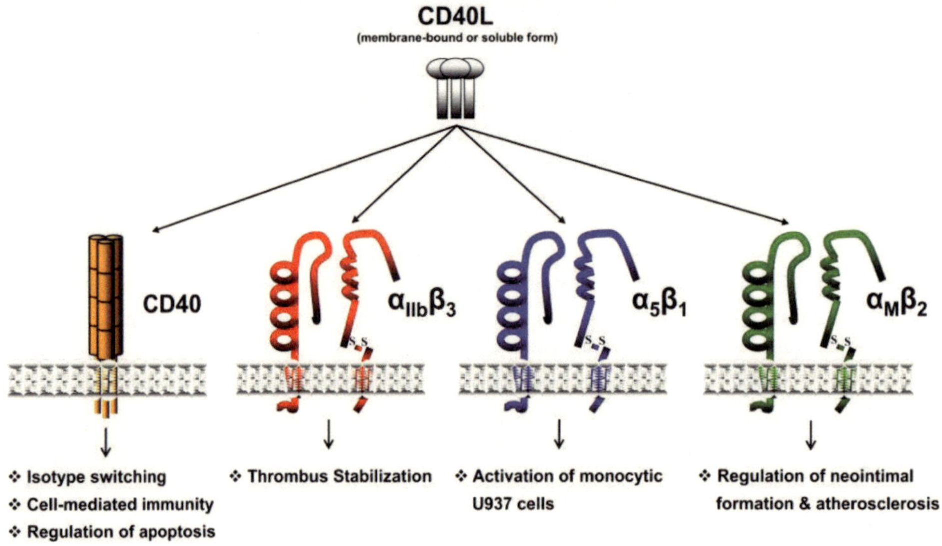

Fig. 1. CD40L and its receptors. The binding of CD40L to its classical CD40 counterreceptor regulates numerous critical biological responses. These mainly include B-cell dependent isotype switching, cell-mediated immunity (production of cytokines, chemokines, adhesion molecules, growth factors, MMPs and procoagulants) and apoptosis. The CD40L/CD40 interaction is at the forefront of the pathogenesis of multiple inflammatory disorders, including atherothrombosis. The interaction of CD40L with the αIIbβ3 platelet integrin is involved in thrombus stabilization and may provide a novel outside-in signaling pathway by which platelets can be activated. CD40L can also bind to the inactive conformation α5β1 and this interaction was shown to induce activation of the human monocytic U937 cell line. Finally, αMβ2 can mediate CD40L-dependent inflammatory responses, in particular leukocyte adhesion and neointimal formation. The pathophysiological relevance of these novel CD40L-mediated interactions in inflammation remains elusive and additional studies will be required to address this issue.

αIIbβ3

The αIIbβ3 integrin is the most abundant receptor of the surface of platelets and mediates platelet adhesion and aggregation. Like all molecules of the integrin family, it will change conformation upon inside-out cellular activation, thereby allowing binding to its natural ligands (fibrinogen, fibronectin, vWF...).[47] These ligands contain KGD sequences and binding is mediated through the KGD recognition domain present on the αIIbβ3 molecule. Interestingly, CD40L also contains a KGD sequence making its interaction with αIIbβ3 possible. Binding of CD40L to αIIbβ3 was shown to induce phosphorylation of tyrosine residues within the cytoplasmic domain of the β3 subunit and appears essential for thrombus stabilization *in vivo*.[48, 49] Indeed, CD40L$^{-/-}$ mice exhibit unstable thrombi, which can be overcome by infusion of wild type recombinant human CD40L and not CD40L specifically mutated at the site of interaction with αIIbβ3.[48]

α5β1

The *α5β1* integrin was also shown to act as a CD40L receptor.[50] Indeed, sCD40L can bind and activate cells of the undifferentiated human monocytic U937 cell line in a CD40- and αIIbβ3-independent manner. Binding to this cell line was reversed by an anti-*α5β1* antibody, as well as in the presence of soluble *α5β1*, thus confirming *α5β1* specificity. Moreover, this interaction is unaffected by pre-treatment of CD40L with soluble CD40, indicating that CD40L can bind both CD40 and *α5β1* concomitantly.[50] Interestingly, CD40L binds to inactive *α5β1*, contrary to most ligands of the integrin family. However, the physiological relevance of this interaction remains unexplored and additional studies are needed to fully characterize the interplay that might take place between CD40L and *α5β1* in inflammatory disorders.

αMβ2

The αMβ2 (Mac-1) integrin mediates firm adhesion of leukocytes to inflamed vessels by interacting with its endothelial cell counterreceptor intercellular adhesion molecule 1 (ICAM-1).[51] CD40L was also recently shown to bind to active αMβ2 and this interaction may represent an alternative pathway for CD40L-mediated inflammation.[52] Indeed, inhibition of this novel CD40L binding partner significantly attenuates leukocyte accumulation at sites of inflammation and reduces atherogenesis, indicating that CD40L may promote, at least in part, atherosclerotic lesions in a αMβ2-dependent manner. Again, the relative contribution of this CD40L receptor (in comparison to CD40) in the development of inflammatory disorders such as atherothrombosis remains unknown. Perhaps, each of these CD40L receptors may interfere at different stages of the disease, thus contributing to proinflammatory reactions and atherogenesis in their own way.

3. CD40L in atherothrombosis

The involvement of CD40L in the pathogenesis of atherothrombosis is supported by numerous studies. Targeting of CD40L by both pharmacological and genetic approaches has highlighted the importance of this molecule in all stages of the disease. In 1998, Mach et al. showed that treatment of hyperlipidemic LDLR$^{-/-}$ mice with an anti-CD40L antibody significantly ameliorates the size and lipid contents of atherosclerotic lesions.[53] These results were further confirmed by a genetic approach, which showed that CD40L$^{-/-}$/ApoE$^{-/-}$ mice exhibit considerably smaller plaque area than control ApoE$^{-/-}$ mice.[8] Moreover, these animals display enhanced collagen fibrils within the fibrous cap of lesions, a key component of plaque stability. In an additional study, the administration of an anti-CD40L antibody in ApoE$^{-/-}$ mice, at the onset of lesions or once atherosclerotic lesions are fully established, reduces lipid contents and increases plaque stability.[54] Taken together, these studies support the contribution of CD40L in plaque initiation, progression and stability (Figure 2).

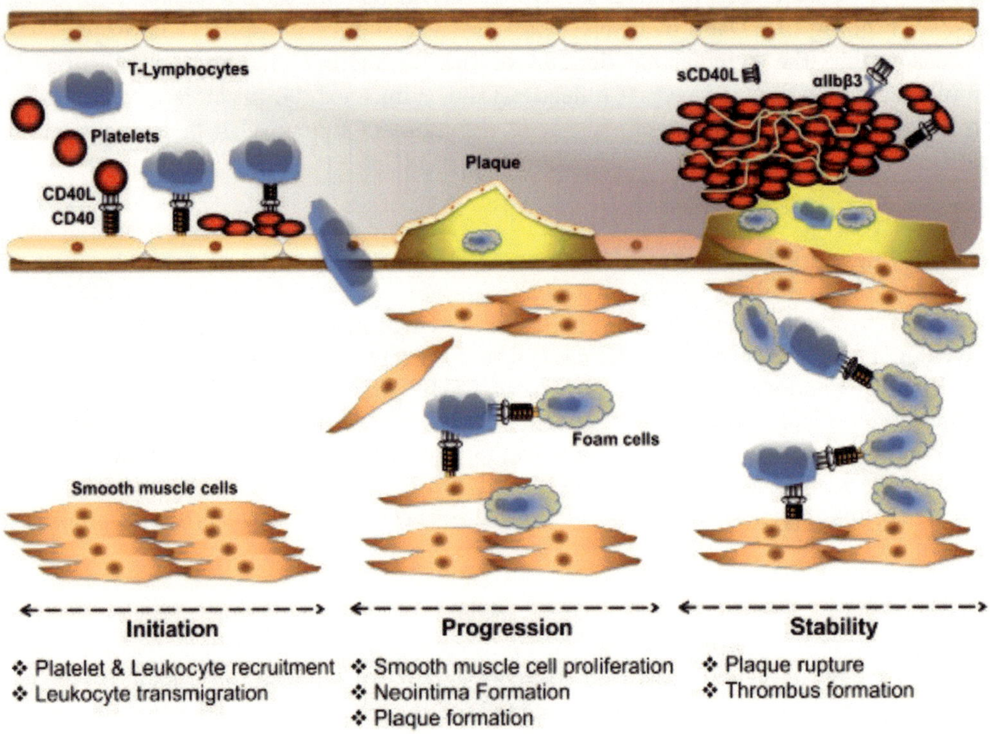

Fig. 2. Role of CD40L in atherothrombosis. The incorporation of oxidized LDLs, among other factors, may upregulate the expression of the CD40L system on the endothelium, thereby promoting the recruitment of platelets and leukocytes at the sites of injury. The CD40L-dependent adhesion of T-lymphocytes and platelets to the endothelium induces an important inflammatory response characterized by the secretion of various cytokines and the upregulation of additional endothelial adhesion molecules. This favors in turn the incorporation and transmigration of additional leukocytes, in particular monocytes. Once in the sub-endothelial space, CD40L/CD40 interactions between foam cells (macrophages which have undergone phagocytosis of oxidized LDL particules), T-lymphocytes and smooth muscle cells take place. These cross talks ultimately lead in part to the proliferation of smooth muscle cells into the intima and promote vascular angiogenesis, primarily through the secretion of key inflammatory and angiogenic cytokines and chemokines. This process eventually yields a stable lipid-enriched atherosclerotic plaque surrounded by a fibrous cap. Plaque stability is threatened by the production of MMPs, which are directly responsible for collagen degradation and rupture of the fibrous cap. The binding of CD40 on endothelial cells, macrophages and smooth muscle cells can provoke the secretion of a long list of MMPs. Following rupture, platelets rapidly adhere to the surface of the highly pro-thrombotic contents of the atherosclerotic plaque, thereby leading to thrombus formation and arterial occlusion. CD40L may also be involved in thrombus formation and procoagulant activity. CD40L binding to the endothelium promotes tissue factor expression, while the binding of CD40L (soluble and membrane-bound forms) to CD40 and αIIbβ3 on platelets enhances platelets aggregation and thrombus stabilization, respectively.

3.1 Initiation of lesions and leukocyte recruitment

Plaque initiation is normally characterized by the accumulation of low-density lipoproteins (LDL) in the arterial wall and the subsequent recruitment and transmigration of leukocytes within the sub-endothelial space.[1] The initial trigger of CD40L (and CD40) expression within cells of the developing atherosclerotic plaque (endothelial cells, lymphocytes, platelets, monocytes/macrophages, and smooth muscle cells) remains elusive. Possible candidates include oxidized LDL, infectious pathogens and alterations in vascular hemodynamic forces.[55-57] For instance it has been demonstrated that lipid lowering reduces CD40L expression in atheroma.[55] In addition, oxidized LDL were reported to induce the expression of CD40 on endothelial cells, which can then bind CD40L from activated T-lymphocytes adherent to the site of injury.[58] CD40 activation on endothelial cells provides a critical proinflammatory signal for the initiation of lesions. Indeed, the CD40L/CD40 interaction favors the up-regulation of adhesion molecules (E-selectin, P-selectin, vascular cell adhesion molecule-1 [VCAM-1] and ICAM-1) and leads to the secretion of proinflammatory cytokines (IL-6, IL-8, IL-15, monocytes chemotactic protein-1 [MCP-1], macrophage inflammatory protein-1 [MIP-1 α/β] and regulated on activation normal T cell expressed and secreted [RANTES]) by the endothelium.[6, 7, 59-62] These reactions induce in turn the incorporation and accumulation of additional leukocytes, in particular monocytes, at the sites of developing lesions.

As discussed above, αMβ2, an integrin expressed on neutrophils and monocytes/ macrophages, has been identified as a receptor for CD40L. This interaction may also mediate adhesion and migration of inflammatory cells at sites of plaque initiation. In agreement with this hypothesis, αMβ2 deficiency attenuates lesion development and reduces lesional macrophage accumulation in $LDLR^{-/-}$ mice, supporting the implication of this integrin in atherothrombosis.[52] However, additional studies will be required to specifically establish the importance of the CD40L/αMβ2 in plaque initiation.

In addition, platelets have been shown to play a crucial role in the initiation of atherothrombosis. Platelets are among the first inflammatory cells at the site of injury and their adhesion to the endothelium provides a fundamental mechanism by which leukocytes are recruited.[63, 64] Because the surface of activated platelets contains a higher density of P-selectin than activated endothelial cells, significantly more leukocytes will incorporate at the sites of injury in their presence.[65] Interestingly, CD40L from activated platelets can also induce a proinflammatory response on endothelial cells, in a similar fashion to that of T-lymphocytes. Henn et al. demonstrated that CD40 ligation on endothelial cells by CD40L from activated platelets induces the expression of numerous adhesion molecules, cytokines, and matrix metalloproteinases involved in the initiation of inflammatory reactions.[16]

3.2 Plaque development and progression

The progression of the atherosclerotic plaque is typically highlighted by the proliferation and migration of smooth muscle cells into the intima, as well as the formation neovessels (angiogenesis), which supports the growth of lesions. This process will eventually yield a stable lipid-enriched necrotic plaque surrounded by a fibrous cap. Once in the sub-endothelial space, macrophages (originally monocytes) undergo phagocytosis of oxidized LDL particles, leading to the formation of foam cells.[66] Thereafter, CD40L from infiltrated T-lymphocytes will bind to CD40 on the surface of differentiated foam cells, favoring the release of further proinflammatory cytokines (IL-1, IL-6 and IL-12), growth factors (vascular endothelial growth factor [VEGF]) and MMPs (MMP-1 and MMP-3).[7, 67] These responses are intimately involved in the proliferation and migration of smooth muscle cells into the intima layer. In parallel, cross talks between smooth muscle cells and T-lymphocytes may also take place, in which CD40 activation on the former initiates a positive feedback loop enhancing the inflammatory reactions already in place.[6] Indeed, CD40 signaling in smooth muscle cells has been shown to induce the secretion of the cytokines IL-8 and MCP-1.[67, 68] Moreover, the accumulation of migrating fibroblasts within the intima layer exacerbates the atherosclerotic lesions in development and the CD40L/CD40 axis might also takes part in this process.[69] Stimulation of fibroblasts with CD40L was reported to up-regulate the expression of cell surface adhesion molecules, thus facilitating their interaction with immune cells at the site of lesions.[70] This interaction also induces their proliferation and secretion of chemoattractant cytokines such as IL-6 and IL-8.[71-73] Hence, the CD40L/CD40 interaction is at the forefront of a plethora of key inflammatory reactions involved in neointima formation and plaque accumulation. Lesions with eventually develop into the formation of a stable necrotic core consisting of infiltrated leukocytes, foam cells, proliferating smooth muscle cells, extra-cellular matrix proteins and lipids.

The formation of neovessels or angiogenesis plays an integral part in plaque progression and several reports have highlighted the importance of CD40L in this process. For instance, CD40 ligation on endothelial cells and macrophages was shown to upregulate the expression of potent angiogenic factors such as VEGF, fibroblast growth factor and platelet-activating factor, in addition to inducing the synthesis and proteinase activity of various MMPs such as MMP-1, MMP-2, MMP-3 and MMP-9.[18, 74-76] These responses are tightly linked to tubule formation and angiogenesis, essential elements of plaque support and growth. Interestingly, the $\alpha5\beta1$ integrin is upregulated on angiogenesis-prone endothelial cells and could also provide a novel mechanism by which CD40L modulates pathological angiogenesis.[77] It would be worthwhile investigating this issue in further details.

3.3 Plaque instability and thrombosis

Plaque stability is regulated by a tight balance between extracellular matrix proteins such as collagen fibers and MMP production. A thin fibrous cap protects the highly thrombotic components of the atherosclerotic plaque. However, upon secretion of MMPs by macrophages and other inflammatory cells present, plaque rupture may ensue following digestion of the collagen fibers within the fibrous cap.[78, 79] This process leads to thrombus formation and may cause complete obstruction of the artery. CD40L mediates several of the processes that set the stage for plaque rupture and its clinical sequelae. CD40L stimulation on endothelial cells, macrophages and smooth muscle cells can provoke the secretion of a long list of MMPs (MMP-1, MMP-2, MMP-3, MMP-8, MMP-9 and MMP-13), the main digestive enzymes of the collagen-rich fibrous cap.[18, 80, 81] Platelets, in addition to their pivotal role in thrombosis, also participate in this process. Indeed, membrane-bound CD154 expressed on the surface of activated platelets can induce MMP upregulation in endothelial cells.[82] MMP secretion and proteolytic activity can be abrogated by physical hindrance of platelet-endothelial contacts, $\alpha IIb\beta3$ interfering agents or anti-CD40L antibodies, thus highlighting in part the importance of platelets and CD40L in this phenomenon.

Following rupture, platelets rapidly adhere to the surface of the highly pro-thrombotic contents of the atherosclerotic plaque, thereby leading to thrombus formation and arterial occlusion.[83, 84] Accumulating evidence also support a role for CD40L in platelet function and thrombus formation, albeit some of the data remain conflicting. For instance, Andre et al. have shown that CD40L plays a role in thrombus stabilization by interacting with $\alpha IIb\beta 3$, while we and others have demonstrated that CD40L enhances platelet aggregation and thrombus formation through a CD40-mediated TRAF-2/Rac1/p38 signaling pathway.[27, 28, 48] Indeed, enhanced levels of circulating sCD40L exacerbate thrombus formation *in vivo,* also in a CD40-dependent fashion.[27] Nevertheless, these studies all support the concept of CD40L as a pro-thrombotic agent, predisposing platelets to enhanced cell function. CD40L may also enhance the coagulation system through the induction of tissue factor release from various vascular cells. CD40 engagement on endothelial cells, macrophages and smooth muscle cells by CD40L from activated platelets or T cells induces tissue factor expression and activity.[85-87] Besides its important role in the induction of the extrinsic coagulation cascade, tissue factor also represents a powerful platelet agonist.

4. Soluble CD40L and coronary syndromes

Given the pivotal contribution of the CD40L system in atherothrombosis, multiple clinical studies have evaluated the association between levels of circulating sCD40L and cardiovascular risk, in particular acute coronary syndrome (ACS) such as acute myocardial infarction (AMI) and unstable angina (UA). These studies can be divided into two main categories. The first type of clinical studies has investigated the link between levels of sCD40L and ACS, while the second has determined the link between levels of sCD40L and prognosis and risk prediction.

For the most part, clinical studies demonstrate that circulating sCD40L levels are significantly higher in patients with ACS and stable coronary artery disease (CAD), compared with control subjects.[88-92] Indeed, it appears that a gradual increase in sCD40L levels occurs with ACS progression, with peaks as early as 9 hours following the onset of AMI or UA.[89, 93, 94] For instance, patients suffering from AMI or UA present with levels ranging from 5-25 ng/mL, depending on the study.[88] Moreover, sCD40L levels are independent from other important inflammatory markers, such as IL-6, sICAM-1, sVCAM-1, C-reactive protein and troponin, indicating that sCD40L may represent a more reliable risk factor, as compared to others.[92] Because sCD40L in circulation almost exclusively originates from the shedding of membrane-bound CD40L at the surface of activated platelets, its measuring levels may reflect a state of platelet activation rather than an inflammatory condition.

More importantly, some clinical studies have evaluated the relationship between sCD40L levels and disease prognosis. In the CAPTURE (c7E3 Fab Anti-Platelet Therapy in unstable Refractory Angina) trial, patients with high levels of sCD40L were 3-fold more at risk of developing cardiovascular death or AMI.[21] Moreover, in the MIRACL (Myocardial Ischemia Reduction with Aggressive Cholesterol Lowering) study, sCD40L levels were an independent risk factor for recurrent cardiovascular events, such as death, nonfatal myocardial infarction, cardiac arrest and worsening angina requiring rehospitalization.[95] Interestingly, individuals carrying the -3459A>G polymorphism on the CD40L gene, are more at risk of developing AMI.[96]

Whether enhanced levels of sCD40L seen in patients with ACS are a consequence of increased platelet activation or a predetermining cause of these complications (or perhaps both) is still unknown. Recently, we have shown that enhancing levels of circulating sCD40L in mice to approximately 45 ng/mL exacerbates thrombus formation in a CD40-dependent manner.[27] This observation supports the idea that increased levels of sCD40L in patients may drive, at least in part, the development of certain cardiovascular complications. It would be tempting to speculate the existence of a positive feedback loop taking place in these patients, where disease initiation correlates with platelet activation and release of sCD40L in the circulation. This in turn could further exacerbate pre-existing complications through enhancement of platelet function and thrombus formation.

5. Disruption of the CD40L system as a therapeutic target in atherothrombosis

In light of all the aforementioned data supporting the contribution of CD40L in inflammation, disruption of this system as a therapeutic strategy for the treatment of atherothrombosis and its clinical manifestations has been investigated. Unfortunately, clinical trials using an anti-CD40L antibody were put on hold due to thromboembolic complications.[97, 98] Interactions between CD40 and CD40L-immune complexes at the surface of platelets have been suggested as a possible mechanism by which CD40L therapy induces these complications.[97]

Since circulating levels of sCD40L result from platelet activation, indirect targeting of the CD40L system through anti-platelet therapy may represent an alternative approach to suppress this important component. Clopidogrel, a potent inhibitor of the platelet adenosine diphosphate (ADP) receptor, has been reported to block sCD40L release from ADP-stimulated platelets.[99] Interestingly, clopidogrel regiment significantly reduces platelet CD40L expression and sCD40L levels in patients with stable CAD.[100] Moreover, $\alpha IIb\beta 3$ inhibitors, such as abciximab, inhibit platelet aggregation and sCD40L release from activated platelets.[101] In the CAPTURE trial, abciximab significantly reduces sCD40L levels and cardiovascular risk in high-risk ACS patients, confirming a link between $\alpha IIb\beta 3$ signaling and platelet sCD40L release.[21]

Statins exert multiple pleiotropic anti-inflammatory effects, in addition to their lipid lowering properties. Several reports have investigated the effects of these drugs on inflammatory markers, including CD40L. Particularly, they have been shown to reduce cytokine-induced CD40L expression on endothelial cells, smooth muscle cells and macrophages.[102] Notably, atorvastatin treatment in the MIRACL trial reduces the risk of recurrent cardiovascular events, which are associated with sCD40L levels.[95]

Most of these agents indirectly target the CD40L system, perhaps through inhibition of platelet activation and the subsequent release of sCD40L. Specific disruption of CD40L or its receptors remains a promising approach for the treatment of atherothrombosis. Although clinical studies using anti-CD40L antibodies have been unsuccessful, alternative targets of this system may render better clinical outcomes. For example, novel anti-CD40L agents that specifically target the interaction of CD40L with its different receptors or inhibition of critical intracellular signaling elements, such as TRAFs, represent valuable approaches.

6. Conclusions

Research over the years overwhelmingly supports the notion of atherothrombosis as a chronic inflammatory disease. Despite the plethora of inflammatory mediators identified thus far as potential contributors to this complication, the CD40L system has attracted a great deal of interest. Besides its pivotal role in humoral immunity, CD40L is now regarded as a key player to all major phases of atherothrombosis, a concept supported in part by the strong relationship between its circulating soluble levels and the occurrence of cardiovascular diseases. In addition to its well-established CD40 counterreceptor, CD40L can also interact with novel binding partners, namely the integrin receptors $\alpha_{IIb}\beta_3$, $\alpha_M\beta_2$ and $\alpha_5\beta_1$. Although most CD40L-mediated functions have been attributed to its interaction with CD40, these novel receptors add complexity to the diverse interplays that might take place during inflammation. The elucidation of the exact physiopathological relevance of these interactions in inflammatory disorders might pave the way for the development of novel anti-CD40L therapeutic targets for the treatment of atherothrombosis and cardiovascular diseases.

7. References

[1] Hansson GK, Libby P. The immune response in atherosclerosis: A double-edged sword. *Nat Rev Immunol.* 2006;6:508-519

[2] Ross R. Atherosclerosis--an inflammatory disease. *N Engl J Med.* 1999;340:115-126

[3] Lusis AJ. Atherosclerosis. *Nature.* 2000;407:233-241

[4] Weber C, Zernecke A, Libby P. The multifaceted contributions of leukocyte subsets to atherosclerosis: Lessons from mouse models. *Nat Rev Immunol.* 2008;8:802-815

[5] Lievens D, Eijgelaar WJ, Biessen EA, Daemen MJ, Lutgens E. The multi-functionality of cd40l and its receptor cd40 in atherosclerosis. *Thromb Haemost.* 2009;102:206-214

[6] Schonbeck U, Libby P. Cd40 signaling and plaque instability. *Circ Res.* 2001;89:1092-1103

[7] Hassan GS, Merhi Y, Mourad WM. Cd154 and its receptors in inflammatory vascular pathologies. *Trends Immunol.* 2009;30:165-172

[8] Lutgens E, Gorelik L, Daemen MJ, de Muinck ED, Grewal IS, Koteliansky VE, Flavell RA. Requirement for cd154 in the progression of atherosclerosis. *Nat Med.* 1999;5:1313-1316

[9] Schonbeck U, Sukhova GK, Shimizu K, Mach F, Libby P. Inhibition of cd40 signaling limits evolution of established atherosclerosis in mice. *Proc Natl Acad Sci U S A.* 2000;97:7458-7463

[10] Davis JC, Jr., Totoritis MC, Rosenberg J, Sklenar TA, Wofsy D. Phase i clinical trial of a monoclonal antibody against cd40-ligand (idec-131) in patients with systemic lupus erythematosus. *J Rheumatol.* 2001;28:95-101

[11] Schuler W, Bigaud M, Brinkmann V, Di Padova F, Geisse S, Gram H, Hungerford V, Kleuser B, Kristofic C, Menninger K, Tees R, Wieczorek G, Wilt C, Wioland C, Zurini M. Efficacy and safety of abi793, a novel human anti-human cd154 monoclonal antibody, in cynomolgus monkey renal allotransplantation. *Transplantation.* 2004;77:717-726

[12] Armitage RJ, Fanslow WC, Strockbine L, Sato TA, Clifford KN, Macduff BM, Anderson DM, Gimpel SD, Davis-Smith T, Maliszewski CR, et al. Molecular and biological characterization of a murine ligand for cd40. *Nature.* 1992;357:80-82

[13] Lederman S, Yellin MJ, Krichevsky A, Belko J, Lee JJ, Chess L. Identification of a novel surface protein on activated cd4+ t cells that induces contact-dependent b cell differentiation (help). *J Exp Med.* 1992;175:1091-1101

[14] Kroczek RA, Graf D, Brugnoni D, Giliani S, Korthuer U, Ugazio A, Senger G, Mages HW, Villa A, Notarangelo LD. Defective expression of cd40 ligand on t cells causes "x-linked immunodeficiency with hyper-igm (higm1)". *Immunol Rev.* 1994;138:39-59

[15] Hill A, Chapel H. X-linked immunodeficiency. The fruits of cooperation. *Nature.* 1993;361:494

[16] Henn V, Slupsky JR, Grafe M, Anagnostopoulos I, Forster R, Muller-Berghaus G, Kroczek RA. Cd40 ligand on activated platelets triggers an inflammatory reaction of endothelial cells. *Nature.* 1998;391:591-594

[17] Karmann K, Hughes CC, Schechner J, Fanslow WC, Pober JS. Cd40 on human endothelial cells: Inducibility by cytokines and functional regulation of adhesion molecule expression. *Proc Natl Acad Sci U S A.* 1995;92:4342-4346

[18] Mach F, Schonbeck U, Fabunmi RP, Murphy C, Atkinson E, Bonnefoy JY, Graber P, Libby P. T lymphocytes induce endothelial cell matrix metalloproteinase expression by a cd40l-dependent mechanism: Implications for tubule formation. *Am J Pathol.* 1999;154:229-238

[19] Schonbeck U, Mach F, Sukhova GK, Herman M, Graber P, Kehry MR, Libby P. Cd40 ligation induces tissue factor expression in human vascular smooth muscle cells. *Am J Pathol.* 2000;156:7-14

[20] Garlichs CD, John S, Schmeisser A, Eskafi S, Stumpf C, Karl M, Goppelt-Struebe M, Schmieder R, Daniel WG. Upregulation of cd40 and cd40 ligand (cd154) in patients with moderate hypercholesterolemia. *Circulation.* 2001;104:2395-2400

[21] Heeschen C, Dimmeler S, Hamm CW, van den Brand MJ, Boersma E, Zeiher AM, Simoons ML. Soluble cd40 ligand in acute coronary syndromes. *N Engl J Med.* 2003;348:1104-1111

[22] Sanguigni V, Pignatelli P, Lenti L, Ferro D, Bellia A, Carnevale R, Tesauro M, Sorge R, Lauro R, Violi F. Short-term treatment with atorvastatin reduces platelet cd40 ligand and thrombin generation in hypercholesterolemic patients. *Circulation.* 2005;111:412-419

[23] Schonbeck U, Libby P. The cd40/cd154 receptor/ligand dyad. *Cell Mol Life Sci.* 2001;58:4-43

[24] Bishop GA. The multifaceted roles of trafs in the regulation of b-cell function. *Nat Rev Immunol.* 2004;4:775-786

[25] Ma DY, Clark EA. The role of cd40 and cd154/cd40l in dendritic cells. *Semin Immunol.* 2009;21:265-272

[26] Dallman C, Johnson PW, Packham G. Differential regulation of cell survival by cd40. *Apoptosis.* 2003;8:45-53

[27] Yacoub D, Hachem A, Theoret JF, Gillis MA, Mourad W, Merhi Y. Enhanced levels of soluble cd40 ligand exacerbate platelet aggregation and thrombus formation through a cd40-dependent tumor necrosis factor receptor-associated factor-2/rac1/p38 mitogen-activated protein kinase signaling pathway. *Arterioscler Thromb Vasc Biol.* 2010;30:2424-2433

[28] Chakrabarti S, Varghese S, Vitseva O, Tanriverdi K, Freedman JE. Cd40 ligand influences platelet release of reactive oxygen intermediates. *Arterioscler Thromb Vasc Biol*. 2005;25:2428-2434
[29] Danese S, de la Motte C, Reyes BM, Sans M, Levine AD, Fiocchi C. Cutting edge: T cells trigger cd40-dependent platelet activation and granular rantes release: A novel pathway for immune response amplification. *J Immunol*. 2004;172:2011-2015
[30] Bishop GA, Moore CR, Xie P, Stunz LL, Kraus ZJ. Traf proteins in cd40 signaling. *Adv Exp Med Biol*. 2007;597:131-151
[31] Pullen SS, Miller HG, Everdeen DS, Dang TT, Crute JJ, Kehry MR. Cd40-tumor necrosis factor receptor-associated factor (traf) interactions: Regulation of cd40 signaling through multiple traf binding sites and traf hetero-oligomerization. *Biochemistry*. 1998;37:11836-11845
[32] Arron JR, Pewzner-Jung Y, Walsh MC, Kobayashi T, Choi Y. Regulation of the subcellular localization of tumor necrosis factor receptor-associated factor (traf)2 by traf1 reveals mechanisms of traf2 signaling. *J Exp Med*. 2002;196:923-934
[33] Xie P, Hostager BS, Munroe ME, Moore CR, Bishop GA. Cooperation between tnf receptor-associated factors 1 and 2 in cd40 signaling. *J Immunol*. 2006;176:5388-5400
[34] McWhirter SM, Pullen SS, Holton JM, Crute JJ, Kehry MR, Alber T. Crystallographic analysis of cd40 recognition and signaling by human traf2. *Proc Natl Acad Sci U S A*. 1999;96:8408-8413
[35] Yeh WC, Shahinian A, Speiser D, Kraunus J, Billia F, Wakeham A, de la Pompa JL, Ferrick D, Hum B, Iscove N, Ohashi P, Rothe M, Goeddel DV, Mak TW. Early lethality, functional nf-kappab activation, and increased sensitivity to tnf-induced cell death in traf2-deficient mice. *Immunity*. 1997;7:715-725
[36] Hsing Y, Hostager BS, Bishop GA. Characterization of cd40 signaling determinants regulating nuclear factor-kappa b activation in b lymphocytes. *J Immunol*. 1997;159:4898-4906
[37] Rothe M, Sarma V, Dixit VM, Goeddel DV. Traf2-mediated activation of nf-kappa b by tnf receptor 2 and cd40. *Science*. 1995;269:1424-1427
[38] Vallabhapurapu S, Matsuzawa A, Zhang W, Tseng PH, Keats JJ, Wang H, Vignali DA, Bergsagel PL, Karin M. Nonredundant and complementary functions of traf2 and traf3 in a ubiquitination cascade that activates nik-dependent alternative nf-kappab signaling. *Nat Immunol*. 2008;9:1364-1370
[39] He JQ, Oganesyan G, Saha SK, Zarnegar B, Cheng G. Traf3 and its biological function. *Adv Exp Med Biol*. 2007;597:48-59
[40] Zarnegar BJ, Wang Y, Mahoney DJ, Dempsey PW, Cheung HH, He J, Shiba T, Yang X, Yeh WC, Mak TW, Korneluk RG, Cheng G. Noncanonical nf-kappab activation requires coordinated assembly of a regulatory complex of the adaptors ciap1, ciap2, traf2 and traf3 and the kinase nik. *Nat Immunol*. 2008;9:1371-1378
[41] Vince JE, Wong WW, Khan N, Feltham R, Chau D, Ahmed AU, Benetatos CA, Chunduru SK, Condon SM, McKinlay M, Brink R, Leverkus M, Tergaonkar V, Schneider P, Callus BA, Koentgen F, Vaux DL, Silke J. Iap antagonists target ciap1 to induce tnfalpha-dependent apoptosis. *Cell*. 2007;131:682-693
[42] Hauer J, Puschner S, Ramakrishnan P, Simon U, Bongers M, Federle C, Engelmann H. Tnf receptor (tnfr)-associated factor (traf) 3 serves as an inhibitor of traf2/5-

mediated activation of the noncanonical nf-kappab pathway by traf-binding tnfrs. *Proc Natl Acad Sci U S A*. 2005;102:2874-2879

[43] Nakano H, Sakon S, Koseki H, Takemori T, Tada K, Matsumoto M, Munechika E, Sakai T, Shirasawa T, Akiba H, Kobata T, Santee SM, Ware CF, Rennert PD, Taniguchi M, Yagita H, Okumura K. Targeted disruption of traf5 gene causes defects in cd40- and cd27-mediated lymphocyte activation. *Proc Natl Acad Sci U S A*. 1999;96:9803-9808

[44] Davies CC, Mak TW, Young LS, Eliopoulos AG. Traf6 is required for traf2-dependent cd40 signal transduction in nonhemopoietic cells. *Mol Cell Biol*. 2005;25:9806-9819

[45] Rowland SL, Tremblay MM, Ellison JM, Stunz LL, Bishop GA, Hostager BS. A novel mechanism for tnfr-associated factor 6-dependent cd40 signaling. *J Immunol*. 2007;179:4645-4653

[46] Donners MM, Beckers L, Lievens D, Munnix I, Heemskerk J, Janssen BJ, Wijnands E, Cleutjens J, Zernecke A, Weber C, Ahonen CL, Benbow U, Newby AC, Noelle RJ, Daemen MJ, Lutgens E. The cd40-traf6 axis is the key regulator of the cd40/cd40l system in neointima formation and arterial remodeling. *Blood*. 2008;111:4596-4604

[47] Parise LV. Integrin alpha(iib)beta(3) signaling in platelet adhesion and aggregation. *Curr Opin Cell Biol*. 1999;11:597-601

[48] Andre P, Prasad KS, Denis CV, He M, Papalia JM, Hynes RO, Phillips DR, Wagner DD. Cd40l stabilizes arterial thrombi by a beta3 integrin--dependent mechanism. *Nat Med*. 2002;8:247-252

[49] Prasad KS, Andre P, He M, Bao M, Manganello J, Phillips DR. Soluble cd40 ligand induces beta3 integrin tyrosine phosphorylation and triggers platelet activation by outside-in signaling. *Proc Natl Acad Sci U S A*. 2003;100:12367-12371

[50] Leveille C, Bouillon M, Guo W, Bolduc J, Sharif-Askari E, El-Fakhry Y, Reyes-Moreno C, Lapointe R, Merhi Y, Wilkins JA, Mourad W. Cd40 ligand binds to alpha5beta1 integrin and triggers cell signaling. *J Biol Chem*. 2007;282:5143-5151

[51] Sigal A, Bleijs DA, Grabovsky V, van Vliet SJ, Dwir O, Figdor CG, van Kooyk Y, Alon R. The lfa-1 integrin supports rolling adhesions on icam-1 under physiological shear flow in a permissive cellular environment. *J Immunol*. 2000;165:442-452

[52] Zirlik A, Maier C, Gerdes N, MacFarlane L, Soosairajah J, Bavendiek U, Ahrens I, Ernst S, Bassler N, Missiou A, Patko Z, Aikawa M, Schonbeck U, Bode C, Libby P, Peter K. Cd40 ligand mediates inflammation independently of cd40 by interaction with mac-1. *Circulation*. 2007;115:1571-1580

[53] Mach F, Schonbeck U, Sukhova GK, Atkinson E, Libby P. Reduction of atherosclerosis in mice by inhibition of cd40 signalling. *Nature*. 1998;394:200-203

[54] Lutgens E, Cleutjens KB, Heeneman S, Koteliansky VE, Burkly LC, Daemen MJ. Both early and delayed anti-cd40l antibody treatment induces a stable plaque phenotype. *Proc Natl Acad Sci U S A*. 2000;97:7464-7469

[55] Aikawa M, Voglic SJ, Sugiyama S, Rabkin E, Taubman MB, Fallon JT, Libby P. Dietary lipid lowering reduces tissue factor expression in rabbit atheroma. *Circulation*. 1999;100:1215-1222

[56] Hakkinen T, Karkola K, Yla-Herttuala S. Macrophages, smooth muscle cells, endothelial cells, and t-cells express cd40 and cd40l in fatty streaks and more advanced human atherosclerotic lesions. Colocalization with epitopes of oxidized

low-density lipoprotein, scavenger receptor, and cd16 (fc gammariii). *Virchows Arch.* 2000;437:396-405

[57] Ruedl C, Bachmann MF, Kopf M. The antigen dose determines t helper subset development by regulation of cd40 ligand. *Eur J Immunol.* 2000;30:2056-2064

[58] Li D, Liu L, Chen H, Sawamura T, Mehta JL. Lox-1, an oxidized ldl endothelial receptor, induces cd40/cd40l signaling in human coronary artery endothelial cells. *Arterioscler Thromb Vasc Biol.* 2003;23:816-821

[59] Lutgens E, Lievens D, Beckers L, Donners M, Daemen M. Cd40 and its ligand in atherosclerosis. *Trends Cardiovasc Med.* 2007;17:118-123

[60] Omari KM, Chui R, Dorovini-Zis K. Induction of beta-chemokine secretion by human brain microvessel endothelial cells via cd40/cd40l interactions. *J Neuroimmunol.* 2004;146:203-208

[61] Pluvinet R, Olivar R, Krupinski J, Herrero-Fresneda I, Luque A, Torras J, Cruzado JM, Grinyo JM, Sumoy L, Aran JM. Cd40: An upstream master switch for endothelial cell activation uncovered by rnai-coupled transcriptional profiling. *Blood.* 2008;112:3624-3637

[62] Thienel U, Loike J, Yellin MJ. Cd154 (cd40l) induces human endothelial cell chemokine production and migration of leukocyte subsets. *Cell Immunol.* 1999;198:87-95

[63] Huo Y, Schober A, Forlow SB, Smith DF, Hyman MC, Jung S, Littman DR, Weber C, Ley K. Circulating activated platelets exacerbate atherosclerosis in mice deficient in apolipoprotein e. *Nat Med.* 2003;9:61-67

[64] Weber C. Platelets and chemokines in atherosclerosis: Partners in crime. *Circ Res.* 2005;96:612-616

[65] Yeo EL, Sheppard JA, Feuerstein IA. Role of p-selectin and leukocyte activation in polymorphonuclear cell adhesion to surface adherent activated platelets under physiologic shear conditions (an injury vessel wall model). *Blood.* 1994;83:2498-2507

[66] Horkko S, Binder CJ, Shaw PX, Chang MK, Silverman G, Palinski W, Witztum JL. Immunological responses to oxidized ldl. *Free Radic Biol Med.* 2000;28:1771-1779

[67] Lutgens E, Daemen MJ. Cd40-cd40l interactions in atherosclerosis. *Trends Cardiovasc Med.* 2002;12:27-32

[68] Mukundan L, Milhorn DM, Matta B, Suttles J. Cd40-mediated activation of vascular smooth muscle cell chemokine production through a src-initiated, mapk-dependent pathway. *Cell Signal.* 2004;16:375-384

[69] Xu F, Ji J, Li L, Chen R, Hu W. Activation of adventitial fibroblasts contributes to the early development of atherosclerosis: A novel hypothesis that complements the "response-to-injury hypothesis" and the "inflammation hypothesis". *Med Hypotheses.* 2007;69:908-912

[70] Springer TA. Adhesion receptors of the immune system. *Nature.* 1990;346:425-434

[71] Yellin MJ, Winikoff S, Fortune SM, Baum D, Crow MK, Lederman S, Chess L. Ligation of cd40 on fibroblasts induces cd54 (icam-1) and cd106 (vcam-1) up-regulation and il-6 production and proliferation. *J Leukoc Biol.* 1995;58:209-216

[72] Danese S, Scaldaferri F, Vetrano S, Stefanelli T, Graziani C, Repici A, Ricci R, Straface G, Sgambato A, Malesci A, Fiocchi C, Rutella S. Critical role of the cd40 cd40-ligand pathway in regulating mucosal inflammation-driven angiogenesis in inflammatory bowel disease. *Gut.* 2007;56:1248-1256

[73] Kawai M, Masuda A, Kuwana M. A cd40-cd154 interaction in tissue fibrosis. *Arthritis Rheum.* 2008;58:3562-3573

[74] Melter M, Reinders ME, Sho M, Pal S, Geehan C, Denton MD, Mukhopadhyay D, Briscoe DM. Ligation of cd40 induces the expression of vascular endothelial growth factor by endothelial cells and monocytes and promotes angiogenesis in vivo. *Blood.* 2000;96:3801-3808

[75] Reinders ME, Sho M, Robertson SW, Geehan CS, Briscoe DM. Proangiogenic function of cd40 ligand-cd40 interactions. *J Immunol.* 2003;171:1534-1541

[76] Russo S, Bussolati B, Deambrosis I, Mariano F, Camussi G. Platelet-activating factor mediates cd40-dependent angiogenesis and endothelial-smooth muscle cell interaction. *J Immunol.* 2003;171:5489-5497

[77] Collo G, Pepper MS. Endothelial cell integrin alpha5beta1 expression is modulated by cytokines and during migration in vitro. *J Cell Sci.* 1999;112 (Pt 4):569-578

[78] Croce K, Libby P. Intertwining of thrombosis and inflammation in atherosclerosis. *Curr Opin Hematol.* 2007;14:55-61

[79] Libby P. Current concepts of the pathogenesis of the acute coronary syndromes. *Circulation.* 2001;104:365-372

[80] Mach F, Schonbeck U, Bonnefoy JY, Pober JS, Libby P. Activation of monocyte/macrophage functions related to acute atheroma complication by ligation of cd40: Induction of collagenase, stromelysin, and tissue factor. *Circulation.* 1997;96:396-399

[81] Schonbeck U, Mach F, Sukhova GK, Murphy C, Bonnefoy JY, Fabunmi RP, Libby P. Regulation of matrix metalloproteinase expression in human vascular smooth muscle cells by t lymphocytes: A role for cd40 signaling in plaque rupture? *Circ Res.* 1997;81:448-454

[82] May AE, Kalsch T, Massberg S, Herouy Y, Schmidt R, Gawaz M. Engagement of glycoprotein iib/iiia (alpha(iib)beta3) on platelets upregulates cd40l and triggers cd40l-dependent matrix degradation by endothelial cells. *Circulation.* 2002;106:2111-2117

[83] Stary HC. The sequence of cell and matrix changes in atherosclerotic lesions of coronary arteries in the first forty years of life. *Eur Heart J.* 1990;11 Suppl E:3-19

[84] Sukhova GK, Schonbeck U, Rabkin E, Schoen FJ, Poole AR, Billinghurst RC, Libby P. Evidence for increased collagenolysis by interstitial collagenases-1 and -3 in vulnerable human atheromatous plaques. *Circulation.* 1999;99:2503-2509

[85] Miller DL, Yaron R, Yellin MJ. Cd40l-cd40 interactions regulate endothelial cell surface tissue factor and thrombomodulin expression. *J Leukoc Biol.* 1998;63:373-379

[86] Pradier O, Willems F, Abramowicz D, Schandene L, de Boer M, Thielemans K, Capel P, Goldman M. Cd40 engagement induces monocyte procoagulant activity through an interleukin-10 resistant pathway. *Eur J Immunol.* 1996;26:3048-3054

[87] Zhou L, Stordeur P, de Lavareille A, Thielemans K, Capel P, Goldman M, Pradier O. Cd40 engagement on endothelial cells promotes tissue factor-dependent procoagulant activity. *Thromb Haemost.* 1998;79:1025-1028

[88] Antoniades C, Tousoulis D, Vasiliadou C, Stefanadi E, Marinou K, Stefanadis C. Genetic polymorphisms of platelet glycoprotein ia and the risk for premature myocardial infarction: Effects on the release of scd40l during the acute phase of premature myocardial infarction. *J Am Coll Cardiol.* 2006;47:1959-1966

[89] Aukrust P, Muller F, Ueland T, Berget T, Aaser E, Brunsvig A, Solum NO, Forfang K, Froland SS, Gullestad L. Enhanced levels of soluble and membrane-bound cd40 ligand in patients with unstable angina. Possible reflection of t lymphocyte and platelet involvement in the pathogenesis of acute coronary syndromes. *Circulation.* 1999;100:614-620

[90] Garlichs CD, Eskafi S, Raaz D, Schmidt A, Ludwig J, Herrmann M, Klinghammer L, Daniel WG, Schmeisser A. Patients with acute coronary syndromes express enhanced cd40 ligand/cd154 on platelets. *Heart.* 2001;86:649-655

[91] Tayebjee MH, Lip GY, Tan KT, Patel JV, Hughes EA, MacFadyen RJ. Plasma matrix metalloproteinase-9, tissue inhibitor of metalloproteinase-2, and cd40 ligand levels in patients with stable coronary artery disease. *Am J Cardiol.* 2005;96:339-345

[92] Tousoulis D, Antoniades C, Nikolopoulou A, Koniari K, Vasiliadou C, Marinou K, Koumallos N, Papageorgiou N, Stefanadi E, Siasos G, Stefanadis C. Interaction between cytokines and scd40l in patients with stable and unstable coronary syndromes. *Eur J Clin Invest.* 2007;37:623-628

[93] Wang Y, Li L, Tan HW, Yu GS, Ma ZY, Zhao YX, Zhang Y. Transcoronary concentration gradient of scd40l and hscrp in patients with coronary heart disease. *Clin Cardiol.* 2007;30:86-91

[94] Ohashi Y, Kawashima S, Mori T, Terashima M, Ichikawa S, Ejiri J, Awano K. Soluble cd40 ligand and interleukin-6 in the coronary circulation after acute myocardial infarction. *Int J Cardiol.* 2006;112:52-58

[95] Kinlay S, Schwartz GG, Olsson AG, Rifai N, Sasiela WJ, Szarek M, Ganz P, Libby P. Effect of atorvastatin on risk of recurrent cardiovascular events after an acute coronary syndrome associated with high soluble cd40 ligand in the myocardial ischemia reduction with aggressive cholesterol lowering (miracl) study. *Circulation.* 2004;110:386-391

[96] Malarstig A, Lindahl B, Wallentin L, Siegbahn A. Soluble cd40l levels are regulated by the -3459 a>g polymorphism and predict myocardial infarction and the efficacy of antithrombotic treatment in non-st elevation acute coronary syndrome. *Arterioscler Thromb Vasc Biol.* 2006;26:1667-1673

[97] Langer F, Ingersoll SB, Amirkhosravi A, Meyer T, Siddiqui FA, Ahmad S, Walker JM, Amaya M, Desai H, Francis JL. The role of cd40 in cd40l- and antibody-mediated platelet activation. *Thromb Haemost.* 2005;93:1137-1146

[98] Kawai T, Andrews D, Colvin RB, Sachs DH, Cosimi AB. Thromboembolic complications after treatment with monoclonal antibody against cd40 ligand. *Nat Med.* 2000;6:114

[99] Yip HK, Chang LT, Sun CK, Yang CH, Hung WC, Cheng CI, Chua S, Yeh KH, Wu CJ, Fu M. Impact of clopidogrel on suppression of circulating levels of soluble cd40 ligand in patients with unstable angina undergoing coronary stenting. *Am J Cardiol.* 2006;97:192-194

[100] Azar RR, Kassab R, Zoghbi A, Aboujaoude S, El-Osta H, Ghorra P, Germanos M, Salame E. Effects of clopidogrel on soluble cd40 ligand and on high-sensitivity c-reactive protein in patients with stable coronary artery disease. *Am Heart J.* 2006;151:521 e521-521 e524

[101] Nannizzi-Alaimo L, Alves VL, Phillips DR. Inhibitory effects of glycoprotein iib/iiia antagonists and aspirin on the release of soluble cd40 ligand during platelet stimulation. *Circulation*. 2003;107:1123-1128
[102] Schonbeck U, Gerdes N, Varo N, Reynolds RS, Horton DB, Bavendiek U, Robbie L, Ganz P, Kinlay S, Libby P. Oxidized low-density lipoprotein augments and 3-hydroxy-3-methylglutaryl coenzyme a reductase inhibitors limit cd40 and cd40l expression in human vascular cells. *Circulation*. 2002;106:2888-2893

6

In Search for Novel Biomarkers of Acute Coronary Syndrome

Kavita K. Shalia and Vinod K. Shah
Sir H. N. Medical Research Society, Sir H. N. Hospital and Research Centre, India

1. Introduction

Coronary artery disease (CAD) and its one of the severe clinical manifestation, Acute Myocardial Infarction (AMI) continue to be significant cause of morbidity and mortality in both men and women around the world. The extent of myocardial damage after an acute coronary event of atherothrombosis determines the prognosis. The diagnosis of acute coronary syndrome (ACS) encompassing unstable angina, non ST elevated myocardial infarction (NSTEMI) (Bertrand et al., 2002; Braunwald et al., 2000; Hamm et al., 2001) to STEMI (AMI) (Alpert et al., 2000), is based on a combination of symptoms, electrocardiographic changes and biomarkers.

The physical examination can be inadequate in identifying atypical chest pain from chest pain of cardiac origin. On one hand 33% of patients with ACS have no chest pain. On the other hand approximately half of patients with acute chest pain, who have the initial diagnostic findings of ACS and are admitted to the hospital, are later found not to suffer from ACS. In the majority of patients with chest pain, the electrocardiogram (ECG) is the most readily available tool for identifying patients with ACS. However, the ECG is also often not diagnostic for acute chest pain and in fact; the sensitivity of borderline ECG for detecting ACS is only 60% (Canto et al., 2000, Panteghini, 2002).

Over the last 50 years, the contribution of laboratory Medicine to the management of cardiac diseases has become increasingly sophisticated. In 1950s, Karmen et al first reported that enzyme released from necrotic cardiac myocytes could be detected in the serum and could be used in the diagnosis of MI. The ensuing years witnessed progressive improvement in the type of cardiac tissue specific biochemical markers and a corresponding enhancement in the clinical sensitivity and specificity of their use.

1.1 Current practice of diagnostic biomarkers in ACS

Today, markers of myocardial necrosis at the down stream of the pathophysiology of ACS; some specific to myocardial necrosis have gained their mark under routine diagnosis of ACS (Table 1).

1.1.1 Myoglobin

The main advantage of myoglobin is early detection of patients with AMI (Gibler et al., 1987, Roxin et al., 1984). The NACB Laboratory Medicine Practice Guidelines have recommended myoglobin in addition to cardiac troponins (cTn) for the diagnosis of AMI patients who present within the 6 hours of onset of symptoms (Apple et al., 2007). The serum myoglobin level rises faster than Creatinine Kinase-MB (CK-MB) and cTn, reaching twice the normal values within 2 hours and peaking within 4 hours of symptom onset. The disadvantage of using myoglobin alone is that it has poor specificity for AMI in patients with concurrent trauma or renal failure.

Current Biomarkers
Myoglobin
Creatine Kinase-MB
Troponins
Natriuretic Peptides

Table 1. Current Biomarkers

1.1.2 Creatinine Kinase (CK)

CK-MB, the specific cardiac isoform of CK can be used in the diagnosis of myocardial necrosis (Mair et al., 1991). This was proposed by World Health Organization and was later extended for monitoring trends in cardiac disease (Apple et al., 2007, 2003). Elevation of CK-MB occurs 4 to 6 hours after the onset of acute MI and remains for 24 to 48 hours. CK-MB is relatively sensitive but less specific as it can be elevated in any conditions following acute muscle injury or in patients undergoing any surgical procedure. Furthermore CK is present in skeletal muscle, intestine, diaphragm, uterus and prostate and thus the specificity of CK-MB is impaired in the setting of injury to these organs. Moreover, serial analysis of CK-MB are required for quantitation as well as qualitative assessment of injury to cardiac muscle, therefore, many studies have suggested that a single cTn can be used as a convenient, cost effective and non invasive method for the diagnosis of myocardial necrosis (Apple et al., 1999, De Winter et al., 1995).

1.1.3 Cardiac troponin (cTn)s

Undisputedly troponin (cTnI and cTnT) are the most sensitive and specific biomarker of myocardial injury (Bleier et al., 1998). The kinetics of both the troponins are detectable in the serum within 4 to 12 hours after the onset of acute MI and depending upon the duration of ischemia and reperfusion status, peak values occur 12 to 48 hours from symptom onset (Apple et al., 1999). The tissue specificity and reliable detected concentration of cTn in the peripheral circulation makes it a good indicative of myocardial injury (Bleier et al., 1998). Moreover, several studies have shown that patients presenting with elevated cTns had a poor prognosis compared to those without detectable cTns (Panteghini, 2002). Because both forms of cTn remain in the circulation several days after injury, it allows for diagnosis even in patients who present very late (Apple et al., 2003). However because of long half lives, one of the disadvantages using the cTn is that neither cTnI nor cTnT can be used for detection of reinfarction after an index event. The other disadvantage of cTnT is that it is present in small amounts in skeletal muscle and is re -expressed in diseases that involve skeletal muscle degeneration. Therefore, an elevated cTn without clinical evidence of ACS should prompt for other possible myocardial injuries, including cardiac trauma, cardiac failure, and hypertension (Panteghini, 2002).

1.1.4 Natriuretic peptides

B -Natriuretic peptide (BNP) and its prohormone N-terminal pro BNP (Nt-proBNP) are neurohormones secreted from cardiac ventricles in response to ventricular wall stress (de Bold, 1985, Nakako et al., 1992). BNP, an established biomarker for patients with heart failure, and NT-pro BNP are elevated in ACS and can identify patients at very high risk for adverse cardiovascular events including death (de Lemos &Marrow, 2002, Ishibashi, 2002). The utility of BNP and NT-pro BNP as markers is based on the finding that it increases in the left ventricle during remodeling after a transmural infarction or as a consequence of previous ischemic damage (Lorgis et al., 2007). However these peptides have poor specificity for the diagnosis of ACS since elevated levels can also be seen in patients with renal failure, primary aldosteronism, congestive heart failure and thyroid disease.

Despite the success of these biomarkers, there is still a need for the development of early markers that can reliably rule out ACS in the emergency room at presentation and also detect myocardial ischemia in the absence of reversible myocyte injury. Misdiagnosis has been reported to be the main cause of treatment delays. Undetected infarctions remain a serious public health issue and represent the leading cause of malpractice cases in the emergency settings. These imperfect strategies resulting in costly and inappropriate management decisions have forced us to search new non-invasive quick strategies in identifying the high-risk individuals. One of them is identifying novel cardiac biomarkers.

Biomarkers have multiple uses in the arenas of research and practice. It is defined as a characteristic that is objectively measured and evaluated as an indicator of normal biological processes, pathogenic processes, or pharmacologic responses to a therapeutic interventions. In clinical practice, a biomarker may be used to diagnose a medical problem, serve as a tool for staging disease, or provide an indicator of differential prognosis.

1.2 In search for novel cardiac biomarkers of ACS

Recent investigations have been directed towards analyzing components, involved in the pathogenesis of ACS, at upstream from biomarkers of necrosis, such as components released during Ischemia, components of plaque destabilization and rupture, factors of thrombosis, components representing oxidative stress, molecules of inflammation and acute phase reactants for earlier assessment of overall patient risk of adverse event and indexing them under "Biomarkers" (Table 2).

1.2.1 Components released during ischemia

The explicit goal is to maintain micro-circulatory flow to prevent even minor infarctions. Only marker that precedes necrosis and permits prevention of the consequence can meet the clinical need. Identifying markers of ischemia even if necrosis is not present may help in identifying a high risk individual who may in very near future experience the consequences of the infarct. The components that have been studied in this group are Free Fatty Acids unbound to Albumin (FFAu), Choline, Ischemia-Modified albumin (IMA) and Heart type Fatty Acid Binding Protein (H-FABP).

Components Released during Ischemia
Free Fatty Acids unbound to Albumin (FFAu)
Ischemia Modified Albumin (IMA)
Choline
Heart type Fatty acid binding protein (H-FABP)
Thrombotic Factors
Soluble CD40 Ligand (sCD40L)
P-selectin
Tissue Factor (TF)
Plasminogen Activator Inhibitor-1 (PAI-1)
Components involved in Plaque Rupture
Myeloperoxidase (MPO)
Metalloproteinases (MMPs)
Cathepsins
Pregnancy-associated plasma protein-A (PAPP-A)
Components representing oxidative stress
Oxidized LDL (Ox-LDL)
Lectin-like oxidized low density lipoprotein receptor-1 (LOX-1)
Lipoprotein-associated phospholipase A-2 (Lp-PLA-2)
Molecules of Inflammation
Vascular Cell Adhesion Molecule (VCAM-1),
Platelet Endothelial Cell Adhesion Molecule (PECAM-1)
Cystatin C
High-sensitivity C - reactive protein (HsCRP)

Table 2. Emerging Biomarkers

1.2.1.1 Free Fatty Acids unbound to albumin (FFAu)

Increased blood catecholamines in association with ischemia can cause increased FFA by activating lipid hydrolysis within the heart and adipose tissue. Apart from this, reduction of FFA use after ischemia can also cause increased serum concentration of FFA. The observed increase in free fatty acids unbound to albumin (FFAu) in the blood with acute myocardial ischaemia has been evaluated for the early identification of cardiac injury (Kleinfeld et al., 1996). Two groups of investigators have preliminarily studied the sensitivity of this marker at patient presentation to the emergency room and have shown that FFAu was elevated well before other, more traditional, markers of cardiac necrosis and had at admission sensitivity of >90% (Kleifeld et al., 2002, Adams et al., 2002).

1.2.1.2 Ischemia Modified Albumin (IMA)

Due to ischemia the metal binding site on the amino terminus of albumin is damaged. The albumin of patient with myocardial ischemia exhibit lower metal binding capacity for cobalt than that of normal patients (Bar-Or et al., 2001a). IMA gained its importance as it demonstrated a good "negative predictive value." In the assay, Cobalt less bound to albumin reacts with the indicator (Bar-Or et al., 2000). Significant changes in albumin cobalt binding were documented to occur minutes after transient ischemia induced by balloon angioplasty and to return to baseline within 12 hours (Bar-Or et al., 2001b). However its presence during ischemia of any other organ and in individual with inherent reduced cobalt binding giving false positive results, lost its specificity for routine use in detection of ischemia (Collinson & Gaze, 2008). However correlating with the clinical conditions and other markers may find its use in identifying high risk individuals.

1.2.1.3 Choline

Choline is a biomarker that is released when phospholipids are cleaved, which suggests that perhaps it could be a marker of ischemia and/or necrosis (Danne & Möckel, 2010). Experimental studies have demonstrated that phospholipase D enzyme activation and release of choline in blood are related to major processes of myocardial ischemia. Several studies suggested that the marker might improve prognostication in patients with ACS (Danne et al., 2003). In a study with troponin negative patients, choline detected high-risk unstable angina with a sensitivity and specificity of 86%. Additional studies are however needed to fully investigate the clinical significance of this marker (Apple et al., 2005).

1.2.1.4 Heart type Fatty Acid Binding Protein (H-FABP)

H-FABP is a low molecular weight protein involved in myocardial fatty-acid metabolism (Glatz et al., 1997). This protein is rapidly released immediately after infarction. H-FABP has been shown in mouse studies to be an early marker of ischaemia (Glatz et al., 1988) (before morphological evidence of myocardial necrosis) and can therefore help with diagnosis of MI earlier (Glatz et al., 1988, C. P. Chen et al., 2004, L. Chen et al., 2004). However, studies attempting to use H-FABP alone for early diagnosis of AMI have produced disappointing results. One review of six studies found that the pooled positive predictive value to be 65.8% and pooled negative predictive value to be 82.0% (Body, 2009). Also it still lacks cardiac specificity as it is found in brain, kidney and skeletal tissue and levels can go up in acute ischaemic strokes and intense exercise. Thus its role as biomarker needs further evaluation.

In a recent study, Bhardwaj et al (2011) evaluated an array of established and emerging cardiac biomarkers for ACS among patients with chest discomfort in the emergency department. In their study neither IMA nor H-FABP detected or excluded ACS. Among patients with symptoms suggestive of ACS, results for NT-proBNP, hsTnI or FFA added diagnostic information to cTnT. In the context of hsTnI results, FFA measurement significantly reclassified both false negatives and false positives.

1.2.2 Thrombotic factors

Plaque disruption and thrombus formation in coronary arteries lead to a variable degree of luminal obstruction to the blood flow and can present clinically as unstable angina or AMI and lead to a sudden death. Three major determinants of thrombotic response are (a) the presence of local thrombogenic substances, (b) the local flow disturbances and, (c) the systemic thrombotic propensity. Thus apart from the local thrombogenic potential even systemic pro-coagulant status may determine the severity of the acute event of thrombosis.

1.2.2.1 sCD40 ligand (sCD40L)

The CD40 and CD40 ligand (CD40L) system is expressed on a variety of cell types including activated platelets, vascular endothelial cells, vascular smooth muscle cells, monocytes, and macrophages. CD40L is a trimeric, transmembrane protein (Hennet al., 2001). Following expression on the cell surface, CD40L is partly cleaved by proteases and subsequently released into the circulation as sCD40L which can be detected in serum and plasma. The main source of circulating sCD40L is platelets (Hennet al., 2001). The binding of CD40L enhances the inflammatory response, acts prothrombotically, leads to plaque destabilization, and inhibits endothelial regeneration. From several clinical studies it has consistently been reported that sCD40L is elevated in patients with ACS and that it provides prognostic information with therapeutic implications independent of established cardiac markers, e.g. cardiac troponins (Heesechen et al., 2003). However, pre-analytical conditions are decisive for the assessment of sCD40L and may preclude routine clinical use (Weber et al., 2006).

1.2.2.2 P-selectin

P-selectin is a cell surface glycoprotein that plays a critical role in the migration of lymphocytes into tissues. It is found constitutively in a preformed state in the Weibel-Palade bodies of endothelial cells and in α-granules of platelets. This stored P-selectin is mobilized to the cell surface within minutes in response to a variety of inflammatory and thrombogenic agents. The mobilized P-selectin is apparently present on the cell surface for only a few minutes after which it is recycled to intracellular space. P-selectin also binds monocytes and neutrophils in addition to activated platelets and is responsible for incorporation of leukocytes into the growing thrombus (Malý et al., 2003). Thus, P-selectin is a marker of platelet activation which in turn is prerequisite for thrombosis (Serebruany et al., 1999a). Fijnheer et al (1997) have concluded that endothelial cell activation is associated with an increased P-selectin concentration per platelet. Elevated levels have been reported not only in AMI and unstable angina but also in stable angina. In our study significant negative correlation of sP-selectin with age in AMI group suggests increased pro-coagulant status in younger AMI patients (Mashru et al., 2010). Its role as biomarker requires extensive clinical evaluations.

1.2.2.3 Tissue Factor (TF)

TF at the upfront of the coagulation pathway plays a crucial role in initiating thrombus formation after plaque rupture in patients with ACS. Tissue injury disrupts vascular endothelium causing its release into circulating blood and hence activation of coagulation cascades. It activates extrinsic pathway of coagulation and act as cofactor for Factor VII (fVII) and initiates cell surface procoagulant activity. It is also known to activate factor X through intrinsic pathway by activating factor IX, leading to thrombin generation and fibrin formation. Since Suefuji et al in 1997 reported the role of TF in AMI, there have been many studies conducted to determine the status of plasma TF and AMI (Kamikura et al., 1997, Nishiyama et al., 1998, Malý et al., 2003, Morange et al., 2007, Xiong et al., 2007) with contradictory findings. We observed increased levels of TF in AMI at presentation (Shalia et al., 2010a). TF exposed from ruptured plaque is the actual trigger but systemic procoagulant status also plays important role. Independent of cellular TF, blood borne soluble TF may play a role in the propagation of thrombosis which also needs monitoring in early atherosclerotic conditions.

1.2.2.4 Plasminogen Activator Inhibitor-1 (PAI-1)

PAI-1 prevents fibrinolysis and thus accelerates thrombus formation. Immunohistochemical staining of coronary artery specimens (Shindo et al., 2001) and mRNA expression studies (F. Chen et al., 2005) have demonstrated increased expression of PAI. While the evidence of increased PAI levels before first AMI attack, was given by Thogersen et al (1998). In our study, increased levels of PAI-1 were observed in AMI patients at presentation and were also more associated with younger AMI patients (Shalia et al., 2010). Hamstein et al (1985) have also reported elevated circulating concentrations of PAI-1 in young men at increased risk for recurrent infarction.

1.2.3 Components involved in plaque rupture

A growing understanding of the importance of atherosclerotic plaque rupture in the pathogenesis of coronary events has led to the identification of an expanding array of markers for plaque rupture. The enzymes that have gained importance in this aspect are myeloperoxidase, matrix metalloproteinases, cathepsins, etc.

1.2.3.1 Myeloperoxidase (MPO)

Leucocytes play a central role in atherosclerotic plaque rupture (de Servi et al., 1996). Myeloperoxidase is a degranulation product, secreted by a variety of inflammatory cells, including activated neutrophils, monocytes and macrophages such as those found in atherosclerotic plaques. It possesses proinflammatory properties and may contribute directly to tissue injury (Eiserich et al., 2002). Its systemic levels predicted future cardiovascular event independent of CD40L (Baldus et al., 2003) and gave in-vitro strong support to the role of neutrophil activation as an adjunct pathophysiological event in ACS that is directly different from platelet activation. Collectively the current evidence supports the need for further studies into the actual role of MPO. One of the important roles of Myeloperoxidase in leucocytes is to activate metalloproteinases that bring about plaque rupture (Zhang et al., 2001).

1.2.3.2 Metalloproteinases (MMPs)

The structural integrity of myocardial Extracellular Matrix (ECM) is dependent on endogenous zinc-dependent endopeptidases known as matrix metalloproteinases (MMP). These enzymes are regulated by tissue inhibitors of metalloproteinases (TIMPs) (Kelly et al., 2008). MMPs may degrade myocardial ECM leading to the development of LV dilatation and heart failure and their inhibition in experimental models of AMI has been associated with reduced LV dilatation and wall stress. Elevated levels of MMP-9 and its major inhibitor TIMP1 have been demonstrated to be associated with cardiovascular death, heart failure or both but not with re-infarction (Kelly et al., 2007). In our study we found that there was significant increase in circulating levels of MMP-9 as well as MMP-8 in AMI at presentation. Moreover the increase in MMP-8 was independent of High sensitive C-reactive protein (HsCRP) and MMP-9 (Shah et al., 2009). MMP-2 is also shown to be elevated post MI (Dhillon et al., 2009) and is associated with poor prognosis (Kelly et al., 2008a). In another study we observed that Serum MMP-3 levels were significantly elevated at presentation of the acute MI as compared to controls (Shalia et al., 2010b) while Kelly et al (2008b) have demonstrated that MMP-3 peaks at 72 hours of MI and plateau levels are associated with increase in LV volume and a lower ejection fraction at follow up. Amongst various MMPs, it has been suggested that MMP-9 may be of value in evaluating patients after acute coronary events (Apple et al, 2005).

1.2.3.3 Cathepsins

Evidence has been obtained for expression in human atherosclerotic lesion of another matrix degrading enzymes cathepsin S, B, K, D and L (Jormsjö et al., 2002). Beside protease function and vascular effects, protease detection and quantization in peripheral blood may help detect atheromatous disease stages and aid in clinical decision-making (Vivanco et al., 2005). Patients with coronary artery stenosis have demonstrated increased serum cathepsin L levels than those without lesions detectable by quantitative angiography (Liu et al., 2006a). Increased serum cathepsin S has been demonstrated in patients with atherosclerosis and diabetes (Liu et al., 2006b) and increased cathepsin D both in plasma and monocytes of ACS patients. In our study increased peripheral blood levels of cathepsin B and K and decrease in their inhibitor cystatin C at the acute phase of MI were observed (Shalia et al., 2011). Moreover plasma concentration of MMP-9; recently identified as a novel predictor of cardiovascular mortality in patients with CAD and also marker for plaque destabilization and rupture demonstrated strong positive correlation with cathepsin B and negative correlation with cystatin C in AMI group (Shalia et al., 2011).

1.2.3.4 Pregnancy-Associated Plasma Protein-A (PAPP-A)

It is known as high molecular weight (200kDa) glycoprotein synthesized by the syncytio-trophoblast and is typically measured during pregnancy for Down syndrome screening. It is pro-atherosclerotic molecule family of proteins; a member of the insulin-like growth factor (IGF) –dependent IGF binding protein-4 specific metalloproteinase (Bayes-Genis et al., 2000). It is thought to be released when neovascularization occurs and thus may be a marker of incipient plaque rupture which was later confirmed in studies demonstrating its increased expression in unstable plaques and their extracellular matrices (Bayes-Genis et al., 2001) and corresponding increased circulating levels in unstable angina and AMI (Bayes-Genis et al., 2001). Interestingly, it demonstrated increase in risk of cardiovascular death, MI or revascularisation even without a raised Troponin (Lund et al., 2003). Evidence for the use of this biomarker clinically remains scarce but promising. More studies and standardized assays will be needed to improve its clinical utility.

1.2.4 Components representing oxidative stress

Oxidative stress in conjunction with inflammation is the one of the important initiators of atherosclerosis. However they also play important role in increasing the severity of pathogenesis of ACS.

1.2.4.1 Oxidized LDL (Ox-LDL)

Ox LDL is involved at very early critical steps of atherosclerosis. Oxidized LDL as well as its antibody (ox-LDL Ab) have been documented to be elevated in ACS patients including AMI and Unstable Angina and were suggested to be helpful in diagnosis of ACS (Zhou e tal., 2006). Imazu et al (2008) examined the relationship among plasma levels of OxLDL, measured by an enzyme immunoassay using an antibody against OxLDL (FOH1a/DLH3) and apolipoprotein B, at the onset of ACS. Plasma levels of OxLDL were significantly higher in patients with new-onset type ACS than in those with worsening type ACS (2.98 versus 1.53 mg/dL, P = 0.002). In conclusion, plasma levels of OxLDL were demonstrated to be associated with CHD and significantly higher in patients with new-onset ACS. The findings of the study suggested that plasma OxLDL can be a marker of the development of ACS. Oxidized low-density lipoprotein (oxLDL)/beta(2)-glycoprotein I (beta2GPI) complexes implicated in atherogenesis were also demonstrated to be associated with severe coronary artery disease and a 3.5-fold increased risk for adverse outcomes (Greco et al., 2010).

1.2.4.2 Lectin-like Oxidized low density lipoprotein receptor-1 (LOX-1)

LOX-1 is a multi-ligand receptor, whose repertoire of ligands includes oxidized low-density lipoprotein, advanced glycation endproducts, platelets, neutrophils, apoptotic/aged cells and bacteria. Sustained expression of LOX-1 by critical target cells, including endothelial cells, smooth muscle cells and macrophages in proximity to these ligands, sets the stage for chronic cellular activation and tissue damage suggesting the interaction of cellular LOX-1 with its ligands to contribute to the formation and development of atherosclerotic plaques. (Navarra et al, 2010). It was demonstrated to be elevated in ACS patients but not correlating with troponins or CK suggesting it not to be a marker of cardiac injury (Hayashida 2005). Kamezaki (2009) in an another study have shown it to be positively correlating with urinary 8-isoprostane and negatively correlating with superoxide dismutase in ACS patients suggesting that increased serum LOX-1 reflect enhanced oxidative stress in vascular wall.

1.2.4.3 Lipoprotein-associated Phospholipase A-2 (Lp-PLA-2)

Lp-PLA2, also known as the platelet activating factor acetylhydrolase, is a monomeric enzyme that catalyzes the hydrolysis of the sn-2 ester bond, preferentially when short acyl groups are at the sn-2 position, of oxidized phospholipids. The cascade of Lp-PLA2 activity may eventually lead to plaque destabilization, increasing the possibility of rupture and thrombosis (Hsieh et al., 2000). Confirming the same, circulating levels of sPLA2 were found to increase not only in various chronic inflammatory diseases but also independently predicted clinical coronary events in patients with unstable angina and documented coronary artery disease (Kugiyama et al., 1999, 2000).

1.2.5 Molecules of inflammation

Although molecules of inflammation may have its primary role as the indicator of endothelial dysfunction and in development of atherosclerotic plaque, its soluble levels have been implicated in various studies to be associated with ACS.

1.2.5.1 Vascular Cell Adhesion Molecule (VCAM-1)

VCAM-1 is not routinely expressed under physiological conditions. Expression of VCAM-1 occurs only on activated endothelium and vascular smooth muscle cells in developing atherosclerotic lesion (Braun et al., 1999). It was demonstrated to be expressed especially in the intimal neovasculature and largely associated with leukocyte accumulation; promoting the binding of lymphocytes and monocytes which further move by diapedesis which release cytokines and enzymes important for progression of lesion as well as rupture of the plaque (O'Brien et al., 1993, 1996). Literature reports correlation of sVCAM-1 with the extent of coronary atherosclerosis with elevated levels in AMI (Bossowska et al., 2003, G ü ray ü, Erbay et al., 2004). Consistent with this finding we have observed highest levels with AMI patients and unstable angina in decreasing order as compared to controls (Mashru et al., 2010). In our study age matched analysis also demonstrated younger age group (<=40 years) of patients with AMI with highest sVCAM-1 as compared to age matched controls and in unstable angina it was more associated with females than male patients. Above observations suggest VCAM-1 to be also as an indicator towards ACS in patients with low-risk profile for cardiovascular risk factors such as age and gender.

1.2.5.2 Platelet Endothelial Cell Adhesion Molecule (PECAM-1)

PECAM-1 of the immunoglobulin superfamily is with wide variety of functions such as platelet activation, inflammation, cell survival, in the immune response and in transendothelial migration of monocytes (TEM) (Muller et al., 1993). It has also been demonstrated to have role in plaque formation and thrombosis (Newman et al., 1990, Mahooti et al., 2000). In our study (Mashru et al., 2010) there was significant increase in sPECAM-1 in AMI patients at acute event consistent with the finding of Serebruany et al (1999b) and Soeki et al (2003).

1.2.5.3 Monocyte Chemoattractant Protein-1 (MCP-1)

MCP-1 is a chemokine responsible for the recruitment of monocytes to sites of inflammation that appears to play a critical role in the promotion of plaque instability (Szmitko et al., 2003). In case control studies, plasma MCP-1 concentrations have been shown to be associated with restenosis after coronary angioplasty (Cipollone et al., 2001). However, in a prospective study on a large cohort of ACS patients, the distribution of MCP-1 values in the healthy subjects and the study population overlapped considerably. However, subsequent studies have shown that MCP-1 plasma concentration is associated with different cardiovascular risk factors, and a greater risk of developing a cardiovascular event in the future (de Lemos et al., 2003, Deo et al., 2004).

1.2.5.4 Cystatin C

This biomarker is a low-molecular-weight basic protein (13 kDa) that is freely filtered and metabolized after tubular reabsorption. It seems that it is less influenced by age, gender, and muscle mass than serum creatinine. There is a U.S. Food and Drug Administration-cleared assay that is analytically robust. Some studies suggest that it is useful for prognostication in heart failure (Sarnak et al., 2005, Shlipak et al., 2005), and ACS (Jernberg et al., 2004). This would make sense as it is well accepted that renal function is a critical determinant of prognosis. In our study cystatin C levels did not deviate much from the controls maintaining its normal levels with normal kidney functioning and demonstrated negative correlation with MMP-9 in AMI group (Shalia et al., 2011).

1.2.5.5 Interleukin 6 (IL-6)

As the prototypical acute phase reactants, interleukin-6 (IL-6) has been the focus of investigations for the diagnosis of ACS. The Fragmin and Fast Revascularisation During Instability in Coronary Artery disease II trial (FRISC) study group showed that the circulating level of IL-6 is a strong independent marker of increased mortality among patients with unstable angina and is useful in directing subsequent care. However, the best timing for measurement of IL-6 for diagnosis and risk stratification of ACS remains uncertain (Lindmark et al., 2001). Alwi et al., (2008) concluded that the IL-6 level in ACS were higher than those in CHD. The IL-6 level 4.43 pg/mL could differentiate the acute condition (ACS) and stable condition (non-ACS) with sensitivity of 89.95% and specificity of 77.42%, and ROC of 0.87.

A study by Kavsak et al (2007) demonstrated that IL-6, MCP-1, and a known biomarker, NT-proBNP were independent predictors of long-term risk of death or HF, highlighting the importance of identifying leukocyte activation and recruitment in ACS patients.

1.2.5.6 IL-10

IL-10 is an important anti-inflammatory molecule with so far contradictory findings in ACS patients. On one hand it was shown to demonstrate more favorable prognosis in patients with ACS (Heeschen et al., 2003) while on the other hand it reflected a proinflammatory state in patients with ACS which suggested that IL-10 is as effective biomarker for the risk prediction of future cardiovascular events as other markers of systemic inflammation (Mälarstig et al., 2008). Extensive study may be required to establish its role in the pathogenesis of ACS and its utility as biomarker.

1.2.5.7 IL-18

It is a member of the IL-1 cytokine family, originally identified in macrophages and Kupffer cells as factor able to induce IFN-γ production by T cells which itself is a central proatherogenic factor. Both increased serum levels of IL-18 and reduced concentrations of IL-10 have been shown to have prognostic significance in ACS. Chalikias, et al (2005) sought to assess whether the ratio of serum IL-18/IL-10 levels has higher positive predictive value than the individual measurement of IL-10 and IL-18 in patients admitted to hospital with ACS. Their findings demonstrated that significantly higher odd ratios were found for IL-18/IL-10 ratio (1.74 95% CI 1.09-2.78) compared to individual IL-18 (1.46 95% CI 0.93-2.27) and 1/IL-10 (1.63 95% CI 1.04-2.56) measurements. Recently Hartford et al (2010) demonstrated that IL-18 levels were significantly related to all-cause mortality, even after adjustment for clinical confounders (hazard ratio [HR], 1.19; 95% confidence interval, 1.07 to 1.33; P=0.002). Long-term, cardiovascular mortality was univariately related to IL-18, and the adjusted relation between noncardiovascular mortality and IL-18 was highly significant (HR, 1.36; 95% confidence interval, 1.11 to 1.67; P=0.003). IL-18 independently predicted congestive heart failure, MI, and cardiovascular death/congestive heart failure/MI in both the short and long term. Measurements from day 1 of ACS and 3 months after ACS had a similar power to predict late outcome.

The data from the PRIME Study, a prospective cohort of 9758 asymptomatic middle-aged men recruited in Northern Ireland and France between 1991 and 1993.demonstrated that higher circulating levels of Hs-CRP, intercellular CAM-1 (ICAM-1), IL6 and IL18 to be equally predictive of stable angina and ACS (all P-values of OR comparison >0.05) (Empana et al., 2008).

1.2.5.8 High-sensitivity C-Reactive Protein (HsCRP)

It is thought that one of the driving forces causing atheromatous plaques to rupture or erode, causing a cascade of events leading to coronary artery occlusion, is inflammation in the plaques (Ridker, 2003, Shishehbor et al., 2003). CRP itself mediates atherothrombosis which is supported by a fairly large body of evidence (Pasceri et al., 2000, Nakajima et al., 2002, Nakagomi et al., 2000, Verma et al., 2002, Devaraj et al., 2003). The benefits of HsCRP testing in a primary setting to screen for ischaemic heart disease is very clear, People are risk stratified based on amount of CRP in blood. There are three groups; less than 1mg/l of CRP is low risk group, between 1 - 3mg/l is classified as the moderate risk group and more than 3mg/l is the high risk group (AHA/CDC, 2003). However, its use post-ACS or -MI is less clear. CRP is elevated post-acute coronary syndrome almost exclusively in the setting of myocardial necrosis indicating the level of myocardial inflammation. In a study carried out by us, we observed a three fold increase in the total HsCRP levels in MI patients at presentation; as compared to controls (Shalia et al., 2011).

Elevated peak CRP in the early phase of MI is related to early mechanical complications, including cardiac rupture, ventricular aneurysm and thrombus formation (Anzai et al., 1997). CRP levels post-MI peak at two to four days, then take 8 to 12 weeks to subside to baseline levels. One of the difficulties with CRP is that it is non-specific and also is elevated in the presence of other inflammatory conditions (rheumatoid arthritis, malignancy, vasculitis etc.). A new assay for Human Pentraxin 3 is now available. Human Pentraxin 3 is an isoform which is secreted exclusively in vascular endothelium and therefore may be more specific to the vascular plaque inflammatory activity (Matsui et al., 2010). It remains to be seen if this biomarker can provide incremental information.

2. Conclusion

Thus, non invasive indicators of separate pathobiologically diverse contributors to the progression of ACS, such as molecules of inflammation, components of plaque rupture and thrombosis, could add complementary information in variety of clinical settings. The role of these components in multi-marker testing, in identifying the high-risk individuals, the pathophysiologic stage of the disease and tailoring therapy needs to be established. The future of ACS management would probably shift from single to multi-marker testing leading to better characterization of each individual case by using a combination of both established and new markers for risk assessment and clinical decision making that will substantially improve the outcomes in patients with ACS.

Growing hand in hand with our contemporary fascination are the promises of personalized medicine, the discovery of novel biomarkers in cardiovascular diseases which has been embraced as a major objective of government, private and industry supported research initiatives. More than a decade of advances in our understanding of the complex mechanisms underlying the initiation, progression of atherothrombosis and its complications has stimulated efforts to identify and characterize new markers associated with this processes. In addition newer screening based discovery techniques such as metaloblomics and proteomics have revealed large numbers of candidate metabolites and proteins associated with this disease for which the function or role in pathophysiology has yet to be explained. The clinical application of cardiac biomarkers in ACS is no longer limited to establishing or refuting the diagnosis of myocardial necrosis. Cardiac biomarkers provide a convenient and non invasive means to gain insights into the underlying causes and consequences of ACS that mediate the risk of recurrent events and may be targets for specific therapeutic interventions.

3. Acknowledgement

Authors would like to acknowledge Sir H. N. Hospital and Research Centre and Rajawadi Municipal Hospital for recruitment of patients and Sir H. N. Medical Research Society for the financial support given for carrying out projects related to this topic.

4. References

Adams, JE.; Kleinfeld, A.; Roe, M.; et al. (2004) Measurement of levels of unbound free fatty acid allows the early identification of patients with acute coronary syndrome. *Circulation*, Vol.106, (Suppl II), p. 532.

AHA/CDC scientific statement on markers of inflammation and cardiovascular disease. (2003) *Circulation,* Vol. 107, No. 3, (January 2003), pp. 499-511.

Alpert, J. & Thygesen, K. (2000), for the Joint European Society of Cardiology/American College of Cardiology Committee. Myocardial infarction redefined–a consensus document of the Joint European Society of Cardiology/American College of Cardiology Committee for the Redefinition of Myocardial Infarction. *Eur Heart J,* Vol. 21, No. 3, (March 2000), pp. 1502–1513.

Alwi, I.; Santoso, T.; Suyono, S.; Sutrisna, B.; Kresno, SB. (2007). The cut-off point of interleukin-6 level in acute coronary syndrome. Acta Med Indones, Vol. 39, No. 4, (Oct-Dec 2007), pp. 174-178.

Anzai, T.; Yoshikawa, T.; Shiraki, H.; Asakura, Y.; Akaishi, M.; Mitamura, H, & Ogawa S. (1977). C-reactive protein as a predictor of infarct expansion and cardiac rupture after a first Q-wave acute myocardial infarction. *Circulation,* Vol. 96, pp. 778–784.

Apple, FS.; Christenson, RH.; Valdes, R.; Andriak, AJ.; Berg A.; Duh, SH.; et al. (1999). Simultaneous rapid measurement of whole blood myoglobin, creatine kinase MB, and cardiac troponin I by the Triage cardiac Panel for detection of myocardial infarction. *Clin Chem,* Vol. 45, No. 2 (February 1999), pp. 199-205.

Apple, FS.; Quist, HE.; Doyle, PJ.; Otto, AP. & Murakami, MM. (2003). Plasma 99th percentile reference limits for cardiac troponin and creatine kinase MB mass for use with European Society of Cardiology/American College of Cardiology consensus recommendations. *Clin Chem,* Vol. 49, No. 8 (August 2003), pp. 1331-1336.

Apple, FS.; Wu, AH.; Mair, J.; Ravkilde, J.; Panteghini, M.; Tate, J.; et al. (2005). Future biomarkers for detection of ischemia and risk stratification in acute coronary syndrome. *Clin Chem,* Vol. 51: No. 5, (May 2005), pp. 810–824.

Apple, FS.; Jesse, RL.; Kristin Newby, LK.; Wu, AHB. & Christenson, RH. (2007). National academy of clinical biochemistry and IFCC committee for standardization of markers of cardiac damage laboratory medicine practice guidelines: analytical issues for biomarkers of acute coronary syndromes. *Clin Chem,* Vol. 53, No. 4, (March 2007), pp. 547–551.

Baldus, S.; Heeschen, C.; Meinertz, T.; Zeiher, AM.; Eiserich, JP.; Munzel, T. et al. (2003). Myeloperoxidase serum levels predict risk in patients with acute coronary syndromes. *Circulation,* Vol. 108, No. 12, (September 2003), pp. 1440–1445.

Bar-Or, D.; Lau, E. & Winkler, JV. (2000). A novel assay for cobalt-albumin binding and its potential as a marker for myocardial ischemia: a preliminary report. *J Emerg Med,* Vol. 19, No. 4, (November 2000) pp. 311–315.

Bar-Or, D.; Curtis, G.; Rao, N.; Bampos, N. & Lau E. (2001). Characterization of the Co^{2+} and Ni^{2+} binding amino-acid residues of the N-terminus of human albumin. An insight into the mechanism of a new assay for myocardial ischemia. *Eur. J. Biochem,* Vol. 268, No. 1 (January 2001), pp. 42–47.

Bar-Or, D.; Winkler, JV.; VanBenthuysen, K.; Harris, L.; Lau, E. & Hetzel, FW. (2001). Reduced albumin-cobalt binding with transient myocardial ischemia after elective percutaneous transluminal coronary angioplasty: a preliminary comparison to creatine kinase-MB, myoglobin, and troponin I. *Am. Heart J*, Vol. 141, No. 6, (Jun 2001), pp. 985–991.

Bayes-Genis, A.; Conover, CA. & Schwartz RS. (2000). The insulin-like growth factor axis: A review of atherosclerosis and restenosis. *Circ Res*. Vol. 86, No. 2 (February 2000), pp. 125–130.

Bayes-Genis, A.; Conover, CA.; Overgaard, MT.; Bailey, KR.; Christiansen, M.;, Holmes, DR.; Jr, Virmani, R.; Oxvig, C. & Schwartz, RS. (2001). Pregnancy-associated plasma protein A as a marker of acute coronary syndromes. *N Engl J Med,* Vol. 345, No. 14, (October 2001), pp. 1022–1029.

Bertrand, ME.; Simoons, ML.; Fox, KAA.; Wallentin, LC.; Hamm, CW.; McFadden, E. et al. (2002). Management of acute coronary syndromes in patients presenting without persistent ST segment elevation. *Eur Heart J*; Vol. 23, No. 23, (December 2002), pp. 1809–1840.

Bhardwaj, A.; Truo, QA.; Peacock, WF.; Yeo, KT.; Storrow A.; Thomas, S.; et al. (2011). A multicenter comparison of established and emerging cardiac biomarker for the diagnostic evaluation of chest pain in the emergency department. *Am Heart J*. Vol. 162, No. 2, (August 2011), 276-282.e1.

Bleier, J.; Vorderwinkler, KP.; Falkensammer, J.; Mair P.; Dapunt, O.; Puschendorf, B.; et al. (1998). Different intracellular compartmentations of cardiac troponins and myosin heavy chains: a casual connection to their different early release after myocardial damage. *Clin Chem,* Vol. 44, No. 9 (September 1998), pp. 1912-1918.

Body, R. (2009). Towards evidence based emergency medicine: Best BETs from the Manchester Royal Infirmary. Bet 2. Heart Fatty Acid binding protein for rapid diagnosis of acute myocardial infarction in the emergency department. *Emerg Med J*. Vol. 26, No. 7, (July 2009), pp. 519–522.

Bossowska, A.; Kiersnowska-Rogowska, B.; Bossowski, A.; Galar, B. & Sowiński, P. (2003). Assessment of serum levels of adhesion molecules (sICAM-1, sVCAM-1, sE-selectin) in stable and unstable angina and acute myocardial infarction. *Przegl Lek,* Vol. 60, No. 7, pp. 445-450.

Braun, M.; Pietsch, P.; Schror, K,; Baumnann, G. & Felix, SB. (1999). Cellular adhesion molecules on vascular smooth muscle cells. *Cardiovasc Res*, Vol. 41: No. 2, (February 1999) pp. 395-401.

Braunwald, E.; Antman, EM.; Beasley, JW.; Califf, RM.;, Cheitlin, MD.; Hochman, JS.; et al. (2000). ACC/AHA guidelines for the management of patients with unstable angina and non-STsegment elevation myocardial infarction: a report of the American College of Cardiology/American Heart Association task force on practice guidelines (Committee on the management of patients with unstable angina). *J Am Coll Cardiol*; Vol. 36, No. 3, (September 2000), pp. 970–1062.

Canto, JG.; Shlipak, MG.; Rogers, WJ.; Malmgren, JA.; Frederick, PD.; Lambrew, CT. et al. (2000). Prevalence, clinical characteristics, and mortality among patients with myocardial infarction presenting without chest pain. *JAMA* Vol. 283, No. 24, (Jun 2000), pp. 3223-3229.

Chalikias, GK.; Tziakas, DN.; Kaski, JC.; Hatzinikolaou, EI.; Stakos, DA.; Tentes, IK.; et al. (2005) Interleukin-18: interleukin-10 ratio and in-hospital adverse events in patients with acute coronary syndrome. *Atherosclerosis,* Vol. 182, No. 1, (September 2005), pp.135-143.

Chan, CP.; Sanderson, JE.; Glatz, JF.; Cheng, WS.; Hempel, A. & Renneberg R. (2004). A superior early myocardial infarction marker. Human heart-type fatty acid-binding protein. *Z Kardiol,* Vol. 93, No. 5 (May 2004), pp. 388–397.

Chen, F.; Eriksson, P.; Hansson, GK.; Herzfeld, I.; Klein, M.; Hansson, LO.; et al. (2005). Expression of matrix metalloproteinase 9 and its regulators in the unstable coronary atherosclerotic plaque. *Int J Mol Med,* Vol. 15, No. 1 (Jan 2005), pp. 57-65.

Chen, L.; Guo, X. & Yang, F. (2004). Role of heart-type fatty acid binding protein in early detection of acute myocardial infarction in comparison with cTnI, CK-MB and myoglobin. *J Huazhong Univ Sci Technolog Med Sci, Vol.* 24, No. 5, pp. 449–451.

Cipollone, F.; Marini, M.; Fazia, M.; Pini , B.; Iezzi, A.; Reale, M.; et al. (2001). Elevated circulating levels of monocyte chemoattractant protein-1 in patients with restenosis after coronary angioplasty. *Arterioscler Thromb Vasc Biol,* Vol. 21, No. 3, (March 2001), pp. 327–334.

Collinson, PO. & Gaze DC. (2008). Ischaemia-modified albumin: clinical utility and pitfalls in measurement. *J Clin Pathol* Vol. 61, No. 9, (September 2008), pp. 1025-1028.

Danne, O.; Möckel, M.; Lueders, C.; Mu¨gge, C.; Zschunke, GA.; Lufft, H. et al. (2003). Prognostic implications of elevated whole blood choline levels in acute coronary syndromes. *Am J Cardiol,* Vol. 91, No. 9 (May 2003), pp. 1060–1067.

Danne, O. & Möckel, M. (2010). Choline in acute coronary syndrome: an emerging biomarker with implications for the integrated assessment of plaque vulnerability. *Expert Rev Mol Diagn,* Vol. 10, No. 2, (March 2010), pp. 159-171.

de Bold, AJ. (1985). Atrial natriuretic factor: a hormone produced by the heart. *Science,* Vol. 230, No. 4727, (November 1985), pp. 767–770.

de Lemos, JA. & Morrow, DA. (2002). Brain natriuretic peptide measurement in acute coronary syndromes: ready for clinical application? *Circulation,* Vol. 106, No. 23, (December 2002), pp. 2868–2870.

de Lemos JA, Morrow DA, Sabatine MS, Murphy SA, Gibson CM, Antman EM, et al. (2003). Association between plasma levels of monocyte chemoattractant protein-1 and long term clinical outcomes in patients with acute coronary syndromes. *Circulation,* Vol. 107, No. 5, (February 2003), pp.690–695.

de Servi, S.; Mazzone, A.; Ricevuti, G.; Mazzucchelli, I.; Fossati, G.; Angoli, L.; et al: (1996). Expression of neutrophil and monocyte CD11B/CD18 adhesion molecules at different sites of the coronary tree in unstable angina pectoris. *Am J Cardiol,* Vol. 78, No. 5 (September 1996), pp. 564-568.

De Winter, RJ.; Koster, RW.; Sturk A. & Sanders, GT. (1995). Value of myoglobin, troponin T, and CK-MB mass in ruling out an acute myocardial infarction in the emergency room. *Circulation* Vol. 92, No. 12, (December 1995) pp. 3401-3407.

Deo, R.; Khera.; A, McGuire.; DK, Murphy SA.; Meo Neto Jde, P.; Morrow, DA.; et al, (2004). Association among plasma levels of monocyte chemoattractant protein-1, traditional cardiovascular risk factors, and subclinical atherosclerosis. *J Am Coll Cardiol.* Vol. 44, No. 9, (November 2004), pp.1812-1818.

Devaraj, S.; Xu, DY. & Jialal I. (2003). C-reactive protein increases plasminogen activator inhibitor-1 expression and activity in human aortic endothelial cells: implications for the metabolic syndrome and atherothrombosis. *Circulation,* Vol. 107, No. 3, (January 2003), pp. 398–404.

Dhillon, OS.; Khan, SQ.; Narayan, HK.; Ng, KH.; Mohammed, N.; Quinn, PA.; et al. (2009). Matrix metalloproteinase-2 predicts mortality inpatients with acute coronary syndrome. *Clin Sci (Lond),* Vol. 118, No. 4 (November 2009), pp. 249-257.

Eiserich, JP.; Baldus, S.; Brennan, ML.; et al. (2002). Myeloperoxidase, a leukocyte-derived vascular NO oxidase. *Scienc,e* Vol. 296 pp. 2391–2394.

Empana, JP.; Canoui-Poitrine, F.; Luc, G.; Juhan-Vague, I.; Morange, P.; Arveiler, D.; et al. PRIME Study Group.(2008). Contribution of novel biomarkers to incident stable angina and acute coronary syndrome: the PRIME Study. *Eur Heart J,* Vol. 29, No. 16 (August 2008), pp. 1966-1974.

Fijnheer, R.; Frijns, CJ.; Korteweg, J.; Rommes, H.; Peters, JH.; Sixma, JJ.; et al. (1997). The origin of P-selectin as a circulating plasma protein. *Thromb Haemost,* Vol. 77, No. 6, (Jun 1997), pp. 1081-1085.

Gibler, WB.; Gibler, CD.; Weinshenker, E.; Abbottsmith, C.; Hedges, JR.; Barsan, WG.; et al. (1987). Myoglobin as an early indicator of acute myocardal infarction. *Ann Emerg Med,* Vol 16, No. 8, (August 1987), pp. 851-856.

Glatz, JF.; van Bilsen, M.; Paulussen, RJ.; Veerkamp, JH.; van der Vusse, GJ. & Reneman, RS. (1988). Release of fatty acid-binding protein from isolated rat heart subjected to ischemia and reperfusion or to the calcium paradox. *Biochim Biophys Acta,* Vol. 961, No. 1, (July 1988), pp.148–152.

Glatz, JF.; Luiken, JJ.; van Nieuwenhoven, FA. & Van der Vusse GJ. (1997). Molecular mechanism of cellular uptake and intracellular translocation of fatty acids. Prostaglandins *Leukot Essent Fatty Acids,* Vol. 57, No. 1 (July 1997), pp. 3–9.

Greco, TP.; Conti-Kelly, AM.; Anthony, JR.; Greco, T.; Jr, Doyle, R.; Boisen, M.; et al. (2010). Oxidized-LDL/beta(2)-glycoprotein I complexes are associated with disease severity and increased risk for adverse outcomes in patients with acute coronary syndromes. *Am J Clin Pathol.* Vol. 133, No. 5, (May 2010), pp. 737-743.

G ü ray, ü.;, Erbay, AR.; Guray, Y.; Yilmaz, MB.; Boyaci, AA.; Sasmaz, H.; et al. (2004). Levels of soluble adhesion molecules in various clinical presentation of coronary atherosclerosis. *Int, J. of Cardiol,* Vol. 96, No. 2 (August 2004), pp. 235-240.

Hamm, CW.; Bertrand, M. & Braunwald E. (2001). Acute coronary syndrome without ST elevation: implementation of new guidelines. *Lancet,* Vol. 358, No. 9292 (November 2001), pp. 1533–1538.

Hamstein, A.; Wiman, B.; de Faire, U. & Blomback, M. (1985). Increased plasma levels of a rapid inhibitor of tissue plasminogen activator in young survivors of myocardial infarction. *N Engl J Med,* Vol. 313: No. 25, (December 1985),pp. 1557-1563.

Hartford, M.; Wiklund, O.; Hultén, LM.; Persson, A.; Karlsson, T.; Herlitz, J.; et al . (2010). Interleukin-18 as a predictor of future events in patients with acute coronary syndromes. *Arterioscler Thromb Vasc Biol,* Vol. 30, No. 10, pp. 2039-2046.

Hayashida, K.; Kume, N.; Murase, T.; Minami, M.; Nak-agawa, D.; Inada, T.; et al. (2005). Serum soluble lectin-like oxidized low-density lipoprotein receptor-1 levels are elevated in acute coronary syndrome: a novel marker for early diagnosis. *Circulation,* Vol. 112, No. 6, (August 2005), pp. 812-818.

Heeschen, C.; Dimmeler, S.; Hamm, CW.; van den Brand, MJ.; Boersma, E.; Zeiher, AM.; et al. (2003). Soluble CD40 ligand in acute coronary syndromes. *N Engl J Med,* Vol. 348, No. 12, (March 2003), pp. 1104- 1011.

Heeschen, C.; Dimmeler, S.; Hamm, CW.; Fichtlscherer, S.; Boersma, E.; Simoons, ML.; Zeiher, AM.; CAPTURE Study Investigators. (2003). Serum level of the antiinflammatory cytokine interleukin-10 is an important prognostic determinant in patients with acute coronary syndromes. *Circulation,* Vol. 107, No. 16, (April 2003), pp. 2109-2114.

Henn, V.; Steinbach, S.; Buchner, K.; Presek, P. & Kroczek, RA. (2001). The inflammatory action of CD40 ligand (CD154) expressed on activated human platelets is temporally limited by coexpressed CD40. *Blood,* Vol. 98, No. 4, (August 2001), pp. 1047-1054.

Hsieh, CC.; Yen, MH.; Liu, HW.; Lau, YT. (2000). Lysophosphatidylcholine induces apoptotic and non-apoptotic death in vascular smooth muscle cells: in comparison with oxidized LDL. *Atherosclerosis.* Vol. 151, No. 2, (August 2000), pp. 481–491.

Imazu, M.; Ono, K.; Tadehara, F.; Kajiwara, K.; Yamamoto, H.; Sumii, K.; et al.(2008). Plasma levels of oxidized low density lipoprotein are associated with stable angina pectoris and modalities of acute coronary syndrome. *Int Heart J,* Vol. 49, No. 5, (September 2008), pp. 515-524.

Ishibashi, Y. (2002). New insights into the mechanism of the elevation of plasma brain natriuretic polypeptide levels in patients with left ventricular hypertrophy. *Can J Cardiol* , Vol. 18, No. 12, (December 2002), pp. 1294–1300.

Jernberg, T.; Lindahl, B.; James, S.; Larsson, A.; Hansson, LO. & Wallentin L. (2004). Cystatin C: a novel predictor of outcome in suspected or confirmed non-ST-elevation acute coronary syndrome. *Circulation,* Vol. 110, No. 16, (October 2004), pp. 2342–2348.

Jormsjö, S.; Wuttge, DM.; Sirsjö, A.; Whatling, C.; Hamsten, A.; Stemme, S. et al. (2002). Differential expression of cysteine and aspartic protease during progression of atherosclerosis in apolipoprotein E-defiecient mice, *Am J Pathol,* Vol. 161, No. 3, (September 2002), pp. 939-945.

Kamezaki, F.; Yamashita, K.; Tasaki, H.; Kume, N.; Mitsuoka, H.; Kita, T.; et al. (2009). Serum soluble lectin-like oxidized low-density lipoprotein receptor-1 correlates with oxidative stress markers in stable coronary artery disease. *Int J Cardiol,* Vol. 134, No. 2, (May 2009), pp. 285-287.

Kamikura, Y.; Wada, H.; Yamada, A.; Shimura, M.; Hivoyama, K.; Shiku H.; et al. (1997). Increased tissue factor pathway inhibitor in patients with acute myocardial infarction. *Am J Hematol,* Vol 55, No. 4 (August 1997), pp. 183-187.

Karmen, A.; Wroblewski, F. & LaDue, JS. (1955). Transaminase activity in human blood. *J. Clin. Invest,* Vol. 34, No. 1, (January 1955), pp. 126– 133.

Kavsak, PA.; Ko ,DT.; Newman, AM.; Palomaki, GE.; Lustig, V.; MacRae, AR.; Jaffe, AS. (2007). Risk stratification for heart failure and death in an acute coronary syndrome population using inflammatory cytokines and N-terminal pro-brain natriuretic peptide. Clin Chem, Vol. 53, No. 12, (December 2007), pp. 2112-2118.

Kelly, D.; Cockerill, G.; Ng, LL.; Thompson, M.; Khan, S.; Samani, NJ. et al. (2007). Plasma matrix metalloproteinase-9 and left ventricular remodellingafter acute myocardial infarction in man: a prospective cohort study. *Eur Heart J*, Vol. 28, No. 6, (March 2007), pp. 711-718.

Kelly, D.; Khan, SQ.; Thompson, M.; Cockerill, G.; Ng LL.; Samani, N. & Squire IB. (2008a). Plasma tissue inhibitor of metalloproteinase-1 and matrix metalloproteinase-9: novel indicators of left ventricular remodeling and prognosis after acute myocardial infarction. *Eur Heart J*, Vol. 29, No. 17, (September 2008), pp. 2116-2124.

Kelly, D.; Khan, S.; Cockerill, G.; Ng LL.; Thompson, M.; Samani, NJ. & Squire, IB. (2008b). Circulating stromelysin-1 (MMP-3): a novel predictor of LV dysfunction, remodelling and all-cause mortality after acute myocardial infarction. *Eur J Heart Fail*, Vol. 10, No. 2, (February 2008), pp. 133-139.

Kleinfeld, AM.; Prothro, D.; Brown, DL.; Davis, RC.; Richieri, GV. & DeMaria A. (1996). Increases in serum unbound free fatty acid levels following coronary angioplasty. *Am. J. Cardiol*, Vol. 78, No. 12, (December 1996), pp. 1350–1354.

Kleinfeld, AM.; Kleinfeld, KJ. & Adams JE. (2002). Serum levels of unbound free fatty acids reveal high sensitivity for early detection of acute myocardial infarction in patient samples from the TIMI II trial. *J. Am. Coll. Cardiol*, Vol. 39, pp. 312A.

Kugiyama, K.; Ota, Y.; Sugiyama, S.; Kawano, H.; Doi, H.; Soejima, H.; et al. (2000). Prognostic value of plasma levels of secretory type II phospholipase A2 in patients with unstable angina pectoris. *Am J Cardiol*, Vol. 86, No. 7, (October 2000), pp. 718–722.

Kugiyama, K.; Ota, Y.; Takazoe, K.; Moriyama, Y.; Kawano, H.; Miyao, Y.; et al. (1999). Circulating levels of secretory type II phospholipase A2 predict coronary events in patients with coronary artery disease. *Circulation*, Vol. 100, No. 12, (September 1999), pp.1280–1284.

Lindmark, E.; Diderholm, E.; Wallentin, L.; Siegbahn, A. (2001). Relationship between interleukin 6 and mortality in patients with unstable coronary artery disease: effects of an early invasive or noninvasive strategy. *JAMA*, Vol. 286, No. 17, (November 2001), pp. 2107-2113.

Liu, J.; Sukhova, GK.; Yang, JT.; Sun, J.; Ma, L.; Ren, A. et al. (2006a). Cathepsin L expression and regulation in human abdominal aortic aneurysm, atherosclerosis and vascular cells. *Atherosclerosis*, Vol. 184, pp. No. 2, (February 2006), pp. 302-311.

Liu, J.; Ma, L.; Yang, J.; Ren, A.; Sun, Z.; Yan, G.; et al. (2006b). Increased serum cathepsin S in patients with atherosclerosis and diabetes. *Atherosclerosis*, Vol. 186, No. 2, (Jun 2006), pp.411-419.

Lorgis, L.; Zeller, M.; Dentan, G.; Sicard P.; Jolak, M. & L'Huillier I. (2007). High levels of N-terminal pro B- type natriuretic peptide is associated with ST resolution failure after reperfusion for acute myocardial infarction. An Int J Med, Vol. 100, No. 4, (April 2007), pp. 211-216.

Lund, J.; Qin, QP.; Ilva, T.; Pettersson, K.; Voipio-Pulkki, LM.; Porela, P.; et al. (2003). Circulating pregnancy-associated plasma protein-A predicts outcome in patients with acute coronary syndrome but no troponin I elevation. *Circulation*, Vol. 108, No. 16, (October 2003), pp. 1924–26.

Mahooti, S.; Graesser, D.; Patil, S.; Newman, P.; Duncan, G.; Mak T.; et al. (2000). PECAM-1 (CD31) expression modulates bleeding time in vivo. *Am J pathol*, Vol. 157, No. 1, (July 2000), pp. 75 -81.

Mair, J.; Artner-Dworzak, E. & Lechlertner, O.(1991). Early detection of acute MI by measurement of CKMB mass. *Am J Cardiol*, Vol. 68, No. 17, (December 1991), pp. 1545-1550.

Mälarstig, A.; Eriksson, P.; Hamsten, A.; Lindahl B,.; Wallentin, L.; Siegbahn A. (2008). Raised interleukin-10 is an indicator of poor outcome and enhanced systemic inflammation in patients with acute coronary syndrome. *Heart*, Vol. 94, No. 6, (June 2008), pp. 724-729.

Malý, M.; Vojácek, J.; Hrabos, V.; Kvasnicka, J.; Salaj P. & Durdil V. (2003). Tissue factor, tissue factor pathway inhibitor and cytoadhesive molecules in patients with an acute coronary syndrome. *Physiol Res*, Vol. 52, No. 6, pp. 719-728.

Mashru, MR.; Shah, VK.; Soneji, SL.; Loya, YS.; Vasvani, JB.; Shalia, KK.; et al. (2010). Soluble Levels of Cell Adhesion Molecules (CAMs) in Coronary Artery Disease. *Ind Heart J*, Vol. 62, No. 1, (Jan-Feb 2010), pp. 57-63.

Matsui, S.; Ishii, J.; Kitagawa, F.; Kuno, A.; Hattori, K.; Ishikawa, M.; et al. (2010). Pentraxin 3 in unstable angina and non-ST-segment elevation myocardial infarction. *Atherosclerosis*, Vol. 210, No. 1, (May 2010), pp. 220–225.

Morange, PE.; Blankenberg, S.; Alessi, MC.; Bickel, C.; Rupprecht, HJ.; Schnabel, S.; et al. (2007). Prognostic value of plasma tissue factor and tissue factor pathway inhibitor for cardiovascular death in patients with coronary artery disease: The AtheroGene Study. *J Thromb Hemost*, Vol. 5, No. 3, (March 2007), pp. 475-482.

Muller, WA.; Weigl, SA.; Deng, X Philips. (1993). PECAM-1 is required for transendothelial migration of leukocytes. *J Exp Med*, Vol. 178, No. 2, (August 1993), pp. 449-460.

Nakagomi, A.; Freedman, SB. & Geczy CL. (2000). Interferon-gamma and lipopolysaccharide potentiate monocyte tissue factor induction by C-reactive protein: relationship with age, sex, and hormone replacement treatment. *Circulation*, Vol.101, No. 15, (April 2000), 1785–1791.

Nakajima, T.; Schulte, S.; Warrington, KJ.; Kopecky, SL.; Frye, RL.; Goronzy, JJ. & Weyand, CM. (2002). T-cell-mediated lysis of endothelial cells in acute coronary syndromes. *Circulation*, Vol. 105, No. 5, (February 2002), pp. 570–575.

Nakao, K.; Ogawa, Y.; Suga, SI. & Imura, H. (1992). Molecular biology and biochemistry of the natriuretic peptide system. I: Natriuretic peptides. *J Hypertens*, Vol. 10, No. 9, (September 1992), pp. 907–912.

Navarra, T.; Del Turco, S.; Berti, S.; Basta, G. (2010). The Lectin-Like Oxidized Low-Density Lipoprotein Receptor-1 and its Soluble Form: Cardiovascular Implications. *J Atheroscler Thromb*, Vol. 17, No. 4: (April 2010), pp. 317-331.

Newman, PJ.; Berndt, MC.; Gorski, J.; White, GC.; 2nd, Lyman, S.; Paddock, C.; et al. (1990). PECAM-1 (CD31) cloning and relation tp adhesion molecules of the immunoglobulin gene supefamily. *Science,* Vol. 247, No. 4947, (March 1990), pp. 1219-222.

Nishiyama, K.; Ogawa, H.; Yasue, H.; Soejima, H.; Misumi, K.; Takazoe, K.; et al. (1998). Simultaneous elevation of the levels of circulating monocyte chemoattractant protein-1 and tissue factor in acute coronary syndromes. *Jpn Circ J,* Vol. 62, No. 9, (September 1998), pp. 710-712.

O'Brien, KD.; Allen, MD.; McDonald, TO.; Chait, A.; Harlan, JM.; Fishbe, D.;, et al. (1993). Vascular cell adhesion molecule-1 is expressed in human coronary atherosclerotic plaques. Implications for the mode of progression of advanced coronary atherosclerosis. *J Clin Invest,* Vol. 92, No. 2, (August 1993) 945-951.

O'Brien, KD.; McDonald, TO.; Chait, A.; Allen, MD. & Alpers, CE. (1996). Neovascular expression of E-selectin, intercellular adhesion molecule-1, and vascular cell adhesion molecule-1 in human atherosclerosis and their relation to intimal leukocyte content. *Circulation,* Vol. 93, No. 4. (February 1996), pp. 672-682.

Panteghini M. (2002). Acute coronary syndrome: biochemical strategies in the troponin era. *Chest,* Vol. 122, No. 4, (October 2002), pp. 1428-1435.

Pasceri, V.; Willerson, JT. & Yeh, ET. (2000). Direct proinflammatory effect of C-reactive protein on human endothelial cells. *Circulation,* Vol. 102, No. 18, (October 2000), pp. 2165–2168.

Ridker PM. (2003). Clinical application of C-reactive protein for cardiovascular disease detection and prevention. *Circulation,* Vol. 107, No. 3 (January 2003), pp. 363–369.

Roxin, LE.; Culled, I.; Groth, T.; Hallgren, T. & Venge P. (1984). The value of serum myoglobin determinations in the early diagnosis of acute myocardial infarction. *Acta Med Scand,* Vol. 215, No. 5, pp. 417-425.

Sarnak, MJ.; Katz, R.; Stehman-Breen, CO.; Fried, LF.; Jenny, NS.; Pasty, BM.; et al. (2005). Cystatin C concentration as a risk factor for heart failure in older adults. *Ann Intern Med,* Vol. 142, No. 7, (April 2005), pp. 497–505.

Serebruany, VL. & Gurbel AP. (1999a). Assessment of platelet activity by measuring platelet derived substances in plasma from patients with acute myocardial infarction: surprising lesions from the GUSTO-III platelet study. *Thromb Res,* Vol. 93, No. 3, (February 1999), pp. 149-150.

Serebruany, VL.; Murugesan, SR.; Pothula, A.; Semaan, H. & Gurbel PA.(1999b). Soluble PECAM-1, but not P-selectin, nor osteonectin identify acute myocardial infarction in patients presenting with chest pain. *Cardiology,* Vol. 91: No. 1, pp. 50-55.

Shah, VK.; Shalia, KK.; Mashru, MR.; Soneji, SL.; Abraham, A.; Kudalkar, KV.; et al. (2009). Role of Matrix Metalloproteinases in Coronary Artery Disease. *Ind Heart J,* Vol. 61, No. 1, (Jan Feb 2009), pp. 44-50.

Shalia, KK.; Shah, VK.; Mashru, MR.; Soneji, SL.; Vasvani, JB.; Payannavar, SS.; et al. (2010). Circulating thrombotic and haemostatic components in patients with coronary artery disease. *Ind J of Clin Biochem,* Vol. 25, No. 1, pp. 20-28.

Shalia, KK.; Shah, VK.; Mashru, MR.; Soneji, SL.; Vasvani, JB.; Payannavar, S.; et al. (2010). Matrix metalloproteinase-3 (MMP-3) -1612 5A/6A promoter polymorphism in coronary artery disease in Indian population. *Ind J of Clin Biochem,* Vol. 25, No. 2, pp. 133-140.

Shalia, KK.; Mashru, MR.; Shah, VK.; Soneji, SL. & Payannavar, S. (2011). Cathepsins and Coronary Artery Disease. Accepted in Indian Heart Journal (2011).

Shalia, KK., Savant, S., Haldankar, VA., Nandu, T., Pawar, PP., Divekar, SS., Shah, VK., Bhatt, P. (2011) Study of C-Reactive Protein and Myocardial Infarction in the Indian Population. *Ind J. of Clin Biochem,* DOI 10.1007/s12291-011-0164-9.

Shindo, J.; Ishibashi, T.; Kijima, M.; Nakazato, K.; Nagata, K.; Yokoyama, K.; et al. (2001). Increased plasminogen activator inhibitor-1 and apolipoprotein (a) in coronary atherectomy specimens in acute coronary syndromes. *Coron Artery Dis,* Vol. 12, No. 7, (November 2001), pp. 573-579.

Shishehbor, MH.; Bhatt DL. & Topol EJ. Using C-reactive protein to assess cardiovascular disease risk. (2003). *Cleve Clin J Med,* Vol. 70, No. 7, (July 2003), pp. 634–640.

Shlipak, MG.; Katz, R.; Fried, LF.; Jenny, NS.; Stehman-Breen, CO.; Newman, AB.; et al. (2005). Cystatin-C and mortality in elderly persons with heart failure. *J Am Coll Cardiol.* Vol. 45, No. 2, (January 2005), pp. 268–271.

Soeki, T.; Tamura, Y.; Shinohara, H.; Sakabe, K.; Onose, Y. & Fukuda N. (2003). Increased soluble platelet/endothelial cell adhesion molecule-1 in the early stages of acute coronary syndromes. *Int J Cardiol,* Vol. 90, No. 2-3, (August 2003), pp. 261-268.

Suefuji, H.; Ogawa, H.; Yasue, H.; Kaikita, K.; Soejima, H.; Motoyama, T.; et al. (1997). Increased plasma tissue factor levels in acute myocardial infarction. *Am Heart J,* Vol. 134, No, 2pt1, (August 1997), pp. 253-259.

Szmitko, PE.; Wang, CH.; Weisel, RD.; de Almeida, JR.; Anderson, TJ.; Verma, S. (2003). New markers of inflammation and endothelial cell activation. Part I. *Circulation,* Vol. 108, No.16, (October 2003), pp. 1917–1923.

Thogersen, AM,; Jansson, JH.; Boman, K.; Nilsson, TK.; Wienehall, L.; Huhtasaari F.; et al. (1998). High PAI-1 and tPA levels in plasma precede a first acute myocardial infarction in both men and women: evidence for the fibrinolytic system as an independent primary risk factor. *Circulation,* Vol. 98, No. 21, (Novembro 1998), pp. 2241-2247.

Verma, S.; Wang, CH.; Li, SH.; Dumont, AS.; Fedak, PW.; Badiwala, MV.; et al. (2002). A self-fulfilling prophecy: C-reactive protein attenuates nitric oxide production and inhibits angiogenesis. *Circulation,* Vol. 106, No. 8, (August 2002), pp. 913–919.

Vivanco, F.; Martín-Ventura, JL.; Duran MC.; Barderas MG.; Blanco-Colio L.; et al. (2005). Quest for novel cardiovascular biomarkers by proteomic analysis. *J Proteome Re,* Vol. 4, No. 4, (July-August 2005), pp. 1181-1191.

Weber, M.; Rabenau, B.; Stanisch, M.; Elsaesser, A.; Mitrovic, V.; Heeschen, C. & Hamm C. (2006). Influence of sample type and storage conditions on soluble CD40 ligand assessment. *Clin Chem,* Vol. 52, No. 5, (May 2006), pp. 888-891.

Xiong, SL.; Wang, Q.; Zheng, L.; Li, JL.; Wen, ZB. & He, SL. (2007). Value of plasma tissue factor, tissue factor pathway inhibitor and factor VII assessments in patients with acute myocardial and cerebral infarction. *Nan Fang Yi Ke Da Xue Xue Bao,* Vol. 27, No. 12, (December 2007), pp. 1821- 1823.

Zhang, R.; Brennan, ML.; Fu, X.; Aviles, RJ.; Pearce, GL.; Penn, MS.; et al. (2001). Association between myeloperoxidase levels and risk of coronary artery disease. *JAMA,* Vol. 286, No. 17, (November 2001), pp. 2136–2142.

Zhou, ZX.; Qiang, H.; Ma, AQ.; Chen, H.; Zhou, P. (2006). Measurement peripheral blood index related to inflammation and ox-LDL, ox-LDLAb in patients with coronary heart disease and its clinical significance. *Zhong Nan Da Xue Xue Bao Yi Xue Ban,* Vol. 31, No. 2, (April 2006), pp.258-262.

7

Lower Extremity Peripheral Arterial Disease

Aditya M. Sharma[1] and Herbert D. Aronow[2]
[1]*Saint Joseph Mercy Hospital, Department of Internal Medicine, Ann Arbor, MI,*
[2]*Michigan Heart and Vascular Institute, Ann Arbor, MI,*
USA

1. Introduction

Lower extremity peripheral arterial disease (PAD) is a disorder characterized by atherosclerotic narrowing or occlusion of the lower limb arteries. In addition to its association with impaired mobility and functional status, PAD is a marker of systemic atherosclerosis and is associated with a high incidence of cardiovascular events such as stroke, myocardial infarction (MI) and vascular death.

2. Epidemiology

Eight to 12 million people in United States have PAD (Allison et al. 2007). Only ~10% of patients with PAD have classic intermittent claudication (IC), ~50% have atypical leg symptoms and ~40% are asymptomatic (Hiatt 2001). Its prevalence significantly increases with age; 12 - 20% of those above the age of 65 years suffer from PAD (Ostchega al. 2007). The prevalence of PAD is similar in men and women; however men are more likely to have symptomatic disease (Ness et al. 2000; Aronow et al. 2002; Selvin and Erlinger 2004; Ostchega et al. 2007).

PAD is a polyvascular disease. Sixty to 90% of patients with PAD also have significant coronary artery disease (CAD) and up to 25% have significant carotid artery stenosis (Hertzer et al. 1984; Klop et al. 1991; Valentine et al. 1994; Cheng et al. 1999; McFalls et al. 2004; Steg et al. 2007). In a study at the Cleveland Clinic, all patients undergoing vascular surgery between 1978 and 1981 had coronary angiogram. Only 10% of those patients had normal coronaries and 28% had severe 3 vessel coronary artery disease requiring surgical or catheter based intervention (Hertzer et al. 1984). Patients with PAD have a 3-fold greater 10-year risk (RR, 3.1; 95% CI, 1.9–4.9) of all-cause death and a 6-fold greater risk (RR, 6.6; 95% CI, 2.9–14.9) of cardiovascular (CV)-related death compared to patients without PAD (Criqui et al. 1992). In the REACH registry, by one year , 21% of patients with PAD had developed MI, stroke, cardiovascular death or hospitalization compared with 15% of patients with CAD (Steg et al. 2007).

3. Risk factors for PAD

Risk factors for PAD are similar to those for atherosclerotic disease in other vascular beds with some variation in their individual attributable risks.

3.1 Cigarette smoking

A strong predictor of prevalent PAD and its progression; it also predicts bypass graft and endovascular intervention failure. (Sapoval et al. 1996; Hirsch et al. 2001; Willigendael et al. 2005; Aboyans et al. 2006). Smoking increases the risk of lower extremity peripheral arterial disease by 2- to 6-fold and the risk of intermittent claudication by 3- to 10-fold (Kannel and McGee 1985; Smith et al. 1990; Bowlin et al. 1994; Meijer et al. 1998). 80% of patients with PAD have a smoking history (Smith et al. 1990; Meijer et al. 1998). Interestingly, cigarette smoking is a stronger risk factor for PAD than for CAD with smoker's having a 2 to 3 times greater likelihood of developing PAD than CAD (Hirsch et al. 2001). It is also an independent predictor of the risk for unplanned urgent revascularization of the lower extremities following initial successful treatment (Shamma et al. 2003). With an increasing number of pack years, there is an increase in severity of disease, increased risk of amputation, peripheral graft occlusion and overall mortality.

3.2 Diabetes Mellitus (DM)

The risk of prevalent PAD doubles in the setting of impaired glucose tolerance (Beckman et al. 2002) and increases by 2 to 4 fold in patients with overt diabetes mellitus. PAD presents at an earlier age in diabetics; the prevalence of PAD is ~ 20% in diabetic patients older than 40 years and increases to ~30% among those older than 50 years (Hirsch et al. 2001; 2003). Diabetics tend to have more severe degrees of stenosis and a higher preponderance toward calcification as compared to non-diabetic patients with PAD (Jude et al. 2001). PAD is more likely to remain asymptomatic in diabetics until very advanced. Finally, poor glvcemic control is associated with more rapid PAD progression, increased risk of amputation and mortality (Jude et al. 2001; Beckman et al. 2002).

3.3 Hypertension and dyslipidemia

Although the attributable risk for these factors is less than for DM or smoking, their adverse impact is clear from multiple studies. Uncontrolled higher blood pressures are associated with increased severity of PAD (Ness et al. 2000; Hirsch et al. 2001; Selvin and Erlinger 2004; Ostchega et al. 2007). Elevated total and LDL cholesterol, low HDL cholesterol and hypertriglyceridemia are associated with prevalent PAD (Kannel and Shurtleff 1973; Fowkes et al. 1992; Hiatt et al. 1995; Murabito et al. 2002). The risk of developing PAD increases by 5 - 10% with each 10 mg/dl increase in total cholesterol (Ingolfsson et al. 1994; Murabito et al. 1997).

3.4 Renal insufficiency

Patients with chronic kidney disease (creatinine clearance <60 ml/min) and end stage renal disease have a higher prevalence of IC and low ankle-brachial index (ABI) as compared to patients with normal renal function (O'Hare et al. 2004). They also have a higher prevalence of critical limb ischemia and increased incidence of peri and post operative mortality related to lower extremity revascularization procedures (O'Hare et al. 2003). Potential mechanisms include altered calcium-phosphorus, homocysteine, and lipoprotein (a) metabolism and altered inflammatory and coagulation pathways.

3.5 Inflammation

A number of inflammatory markers are associated with prevalent PAD and outcomes among those with PAD. In a meta-analysis, the odds ratio for PAD in patients with increased homocysteine was 6.8 (Boushey et al. 1995). 30-40% of PAD patients have elevated homocysteine levels as compared with 3-5% of the general population (Hajjar 1993). Elevated C - reactive protein and D-dimer are associated with increased cardiovascular mortality in PAD patients (Vidula et al. 2008).

3.6 Age

The Prevalence of PAD increases with age. In the NHANES study, the prevalence of PAD increased significantly with each decade since beyond 40 years (Selvin and Erlinger 2004) (Table 1). In a German epidemiologic study, 21% of the patients above the age of 65 years had symptomatic or asymptomatic PAD yet again demonstrating increased incidence of PAD with age (Diehm et al. 2009).

Age (yrs)	Prevalence of PAD
40 -49	0.9%
50 – 59	2.5%
60 – 69	4.7%
>70	14.5%

Table 1. In the NHANES study, prevalence of PAD increased significantly with age.

3.7 Race/ethnicity

The prevalence of PAD varies by ethnicity and race. Non-hispanic blacks have the highest prevalence, followed by Mexican Americans and non-Hispanic whites, with 19.5%, 15.6% and 11.7% above the age of 60 years having PAD, respectively (Ostchega et al. 2007). It is believed that these relationships are mediated by a genetic predisposition in part secondary to variations in atherogenic and prothrombotic factors (Folsom et al. 1992; Conlan et al. 1993; Gerhard et al. 1999).

4. Clinical presentation

PAD can present in the following forms (Hirsch et al. 2006):

4.1 Intermittent claudication: Exertional symptoms such as muscle pain, cramping, discomfort or fatigue in the legs which resolves with rest of 10 minutes or less. However, these 'classic' symptoms are seen in only 10 % of patients with PAD.

4.2 "Atypical" leg pain: Exertional leg symptoms which may not always resolve with rest or are not consistently reproducible.

4.3 Asymptomatic: 40 % of patients with PAD have no leg symptoms but most will have some other form of functional limitations.

4.4 Acute limb ischemia: A potentially limb threatening syndrome, classically manifest by one of more of the following five "P's" - pain, pulselessness, paralysis, paresthesias and pallor.

4.5 Chronic limb ischemia (also known as 'critical limb ischemia [CLI]): Accounts for 1-2% of all patients with PAD. It presents as rest pain, non-healing ulcers and/or gangrene.

The severity of symptoms usually correlates with degree of stenosis, adequacy of collateral circulation and level of exertion. Location of the discomfort may shed light on the location of stenosis (Table 2).

Lesion location	Site of symptoms
Isolated infra-popliteal	Foot
Popliteal	Calf
Femoral	Calf
Iliac	Calf, thigh possibly impotence
Aorto-iliac	Bilateral calf, thigh, buttock, impotence
Deep femoral artery	Thigh
Internal iliac artery	Buttock and hip, impotence if bilateral disease

Table 2. Level of disease and associated symptoms

5. Natural history of PAD

Over a 5-year period, only 1-2% of claudicants and asymptomatic patients develop CLI. Nevertheless, the overall mortality rate is 15 - 30% (75% of which is cardiovascular) and risk of non-fatal MI or stroke 20% at 5 years. Patients with CLI have much worse outcomes with an annual CV mortality of 25% and annual amputation rate of 25%.

It is noteworthy that the burden of PAD may not correlate with the presence or absence of claudication. Patients who are more physically active are more likely to present with claudication than those who lead a sedentary lifestyle. Patients who are too sedentary to claudicate may present with CLI as their first manifestation of disease.

6. Classification of PAD

The Rutherford and Fontaine classifications (Table 3) are frequently utilized to classify PAD symptom severity.

	Fontaine classification	Rutherford system		
Stage	Clinical	Grade	Category	Clinical
I	Asymptomatic	0	0	Asymptomatic
II a	Mild claudication	I	1	Mild claudication
II b	Moderate - severe claudication	I	2	Moderate claudication
		I	3	Severe claudication
III	Ischemic rest pain	II	4	Ischemic rest pain
IV	Ulceration or gangrene	III	5	Tissue ulceration (minor)
		IV	6	Tissue loss / gangrene

Table 3. Rutherford and Fontaine classification for PAD.

7. Physical exam

A comprehensive vascular history and physical exam is vital in the evaluation and appropriate treatment of patient with PAD or suspected PAD. Current ACC / AHA guidelines recommend a complete vascular exam (class I B) for patients with intermittent claudication (Hirsch et al. 2006).

The key components of physical exam are:

- Bilateral arm blood pressure (to screen for subclavian stenosis/upper extremity PAD)
- Cardiac examination
- Assessment of the abdomen for aortic aneurysmal and stenotic disease
- Thorough Examination of legs and feet
- Pulse
    - Carotid
    - Radial/ulnar
    - Femoral
    - Popliteal
    - Dorsalis pedis (DP)
    - Posterior tibial (PT)

Pulse should be graded on a scale of 0-3. 0=absent, 1=dampened, 2=normal or 3=bounding. If no pulse is palpable on exam, a Doppler exam using a hand-held continuous wave device should be performed. An absent or abnormal PT pulse has a very high specificity for diagnosis of PAD. An absent or abnormal DP is non-specific due to a high prevalence of absent or anomalous DP in the general population.

- It is also vital to asses for vascular bruits (carotid, abdominal, femoral, and popliteal)
- Other characteristics that may be seen in lower extremity PAD:
    - Hair loss
    - Nail hypertrophy
    - Rapid elevation pallor or dependent rubor.
    - Foot examinations should be performed at each visit for patients with PAD to assess for tissue loss (i.e., ulcers or gangrene) as well as for signs of other foot pathology such as callous formation or neuropathy.

8. Screening for asymptomatic patients

In the PAD Awareness, Risk and Treatment: New Resources for Survival (PARTNERS) study, 6979 patients aged ≥ 70 years or aged 50-69 years with a history of cigarette smoking or diabetes were screened with ABI's (Hirsch et al. 2001). PAD (defined as an ABI of ≤ 0.90) was diagnosed in 29% of this cohort. This diagnosis would have been missed in 85% to 90% had physicians relied solely on patients presenting with intermittent claudication (Hirsch et al. 2001). Even patients with IC infrequently report this symptom as they attribute it to the normal aging process (Dormandy and Rutherford 2000). A German epidemiologic study which included 6880 patients > 65 years of age reported that 21% of these patients had asymptomatic or symptomatic PAD (Diehm et al. 2009). Given that up to 50% of patients with PAD may be asymptomatic, it is critical that these high risk patients are identified so that appropriate interventions may be initiated to prevent the associated morbidity and mortality. ACC /AHA guidelines recommend screening ABI's among high risk patients (class IC) defined as individuals with 1 or more of the following: exertional leg symptoms, non-healing wounds, age 65 years and older, or 50 years and older with a history of smoking or diabetes (Rooke et al. 2011).

The ADA also recommends that any diabetic patient above the age of 50 years who has a normal ABI should have ABI's repeated every 5 years (American Diabetic Association 2003).

9. Diagnostic evaluation

It is necessary to differentiate claudication from other conditions causing leg pain when evaluating patients with PAD. Patients may have an abnormal ABI and present with leg pain unrelated to PAD. Claudication may be confused with pseudoclaudication resulting from spinal stenosis, nerve compression syndromes, arthritic pain or venous claudication. Certain clinical features help differentiate these conditions Questionnaires have also been frequently used for identifying, monitoring, assessing severity of PAD and treatment success. The Rose claudication questionnaire is a simple screening tool for claudication which can be administered by asking 2 simple questions; "Do you get pain in either leg when you walk?" and "Does the pain go away when you stop walking?" If the answer to both the question is yes then the like hood for PAD is 95% (Rose 1962). There is an updated version of the World Health Organization Rose Questionnaire and also the Edinburgh Claudication Questionnaire which are used to diagnose PAD and the Walking Impairment Questionnaire, the Peripheral Artery Questionnaire and the Medical Outcomes Study 36-Item Short Form Health Survey are used to assess severity of PAD and assess response to therapy (Criqui al. 1985; Leng and Fowkes 1992; Criqui et al. 1996; Spertus et al. 2004).

10. Diagnostic tests

Physiological studies such as the ABI, segmental limb pressures, or pulse-volume waveform analysis can help identify functional limb perfusion abnormalities. Imaging methods, such as duplex ultrasonography, CT angiography (CTA) and magnetic resonance angiography (MRA) provide detailed anatomical, but less frequently functional information on limb perfusion. Diagnostic modalities and respective clinical indications appear in Table 4.

10.1 Ankle-Brachial Index

ABI measurement is the universally accepted standard for the initial diagnostic evaluation of patients with suspected PAD and for high risk asymptomatic patients (Hirsch, Haskal et al. 2006; Mohler and Giri 2008; Rooke et al. 2011). It is simple, reliable, extremely sensitive (79 - 95%) and specific (96-100%) and can be performed in a primary care office in < 15 minutes (Fowkes 1988; Lijmer et al. 1996). The ABI is calculated by measuring the systolic blood pressure in each arm (brachial artery) and ankle (dorsalis pedis and posterior tibial arteries) using a hand held Doppler device in a patient who has been resting in the supine position for 10 minutes. The right ABI = higher right ankle pressure/higher pressure in either arm; the left ABI = higher left ankle pressure/higher pressure in either arm. An ABI ≤ 0.90 suggests PAD with ≥ 50% stenosis in at least one artery. (Fowkes 1988; Lijmer, Hunink et al. 1996).

Based on publication of the results of the Ankle Brachial Index Collaboration, a normal ABI range is defined as between 1.00 to 1.40, and abnormal values continue to be defined as those ≤0.90. ABI values of 0.91 to 0.99 are considered "borderline" and values ≥1.40 indicates noncompressible arteries (Fowkes, Murray et al. 2008; Rooke, Hirsch et al. 2011).

In addition to its diagnostic utility, the ABI also provides important prognostic and functional information. The relative risk of mortality increases by 3.1% with a decrease of 0.50 in ABI. Sikkink et al followed 150 patients who were >40 years of age and had ABI< 0.90 and found that the cumulative survival at 5 years was 63% for patients with an ABI of < 0.50, 71% for patients with an ABI of 0.50 to 0.69, and 91% for those with an ABI of ≥ 0.70

(Sikkink et al. 1997). McDermott and colleagues found that poor functional outcomes were associated with lower ABI's (McDermott et al. 2002). Interestingly, functional outcomes did not correlate with leg symptoms, again confirming that leg symptoms are a poor marker for identifying PAD severity.

Resting ABI may be insensitive for detecting aorto-iliac occlusive disease. ABI after exercise should be performed in these patients if PAD is suspected. If resting values in patients with intermittent claudication are normal, then ABI should be repeated after exercise. Incompressible arteries (e.g., elderly, diabetes, renal failure) may yield falsely normal or elevated ABI measurements. Toe- brachial index (TBI) measurement or pulse volume recording measurements should be performed in these patients as they are more accurate in this setting(Rooke et al. 2011).

10.2 Segmental Pressure Examination (SPE) and Pulse Volume Recordings (PVR)

SPE is a physiological test helpful in identifying location of individual arterial stenoses. It is performed by placing blood pressure cuffs at the upper thigh, the lower thigh, the upper calf and the lower calf above the ankle. Systolic blood pressure measurements are obtained at all these sites and both brachial arteries. A difference of ≥ 20 mm Hg between two adjacent segments is considered physiologically significant. For example, a significant pressure gradient between left upper thigh cuff and left lower thigh cuff would indicate a physiologically significant stenosis in the left superficial femoral artery. As with the ABI, pressures may be elevated or uninterpretable in patients with non-compressible vessels. Pulse volume recordings are performed by measuring volume changes in the limb along with segmental pressure recordings (Darling et al. 1972). Segmental pressure examination when performed with pulse volume recordings has an overall accuracy of 90 - 95% in assessing the location and severity of arterial stenosis (Symes et al. 1984).

10.3 Duplex ultrasound

It is recommended by ACC / AHA guidelines (Class I) for routine surveillance after femoral-popliteal or femoral-tibial pedal bypass with a venous conduit (Hirsch et al. 2006).

The 2011 ACC/AHA guidelines recommend that segmental pressures, Doppler waveform analysis, pulse volume recordings, or ABI with duplex ultrasonography (or some combination of these methods) to document the presence and location of PAD in the lower extremity can be used (Rooke et al. 2011). In general, imaging studies are reserved for patients with PAD in whom revascularization is planned, for bypass graft or percutaneous vascular intervention surveillance or for cases in which the diagnosis of PAD or etiology of PAD is unclear such as arterial aneurysm, fibromuscular dysplasia, entrapment syndrome or vasculitis. Imaging studies are also used to diagnose PAD in patients with non-compressible vessels such as those with ABI > 1.3.

Physiological testing such as ABI and PVR are adequate for asymptomatic patients. For symptomatics (claudication or pseudoclaudication) ABI and PVR with or without exercise, duplex or dopler ultrasound are utilised. CTA, MRA or duplex / doppler ultrasound are usually used for patients considered for revascularization as well as for post endovascular interventions and follow ups as well as for post vein graft follow ups.

11. Management of Peripheral Arterial Disease

Guidelines for the management of PAD have been published by

a. American college of Cardiology / American Heart Association which was a Collaborative Report from the American Association for Vascular Surgery/ Society for Vascular Surgery, Society for Cardiovascular Angiography and Interventions, Society for Vascular Medicine and Biology, Society of Interventional Radiology, and the ACC/AHA Task Force on Practice Guidelines
b. Scottish Intercollegiate Guidelines Network (SIGN), and
c. Trans-Atlantic Inter-Society Consensus (TASC) II (Dormandy and Rutherford 2000; Hirsch et al. 2006; Network 2006; Norgren et al. 2007).

Each of these guidelines focuses on management of PAD as a two-tiered process. First and foremost, they recommend cardiovascular risk reduction through vascular risk factor modification and antiplatelet therapy and second, symptom-guided therapy including supervised exercise, pharmacological interventions and revascularization procedures, when needed.

11.1 Cardiovascular risk factor modification

11.1.1 Smoking cessation

Patients with PAD should be referred to a formal smoking cessation program including pharmacotherapy when appropriate. A Cochrane review of 20 prospective cohort studies showed that smoking cessation is associated with a 36% risk reduction in cardiovascular events in patients with known atherosclerotic disease (Critchley and Capewell 2004) and is recommended by all three guidelines(Dormandy and Rutherford 2000; Hirsch et al. 2006; Network 2006; Norgren et al. 2007; Rooke et al. 2011); Smoking cessation is achieved in approximately 5% of patients with physician encouragement and advice along with regular follow-ups and as compared to 0.1% without physician intervention at 1 year (Law and Tang 1995). Success rates are higher with interventions such as nicotine replacement, bupropion or varenicline. When compared with usual care, formal smoking cessation program which consisted of a strong physician message and 12 two-hour group sessions, using behavior modification and nicotine gum had a higher success rate at 5 years (22% vs. 5%) (Anthonisen et al. 2005). Abstinence rates with bupropion at 3-, 6- and 12- month follow up are 34%, 27% and 22% respectively, compared with 15%, 11% and 9%, for placebo(Tonstad et al. 2003). A combination of bupropion and nicotine replacement is superior to nicotine replacement alone, however but has similar in efficacy to only monotherapy with bupropion (Jorenby et al. 1999). Varenicline has been proven effective in smokers with cardiovascular disease including those with PAD. Rigotti et al conducted a multicenter, randomized, double-blind, placebo-controlled trial comparing the efficacy and safety of varenicline (12 weeks treatment) with placebo showed a continuous abstinence rate was higher for varenicline than placebo during weeks 9 through 12 (47.0% versus 13.9%;) and weeks 9 through 52 (19.2% versus 7.2%). The varenicline and placebo groups did not differ significantly in cardiovascular mortality, all-cause mortality, cardiovascular events, or serious adverse events. (Rigotti et al. 2010). Another RCT compared varenicline vs. bupropion vs placebo showed varenicline was more efficacious than bupropion or placebo in short term (9-12 weeks) (43.9% vs. 29.8% vs. 17.6)% as well as long term period 9 - 52 weeks) (23% vs. 14.6% vs. 10.3%) (Jorenby et al. 2006).

11.1.2 Diabetes Mellitus

Approximately 20-30% in patients with DM have PAD (Marso and Hiatt 2006). The severity of PAD in this cohort correlates with the duration and severity of DM (Selvin et al. 2004; Wattanakit et al. 2005). With every 1% increase in glycosylated hemoglobin levels, the risk of PAD increases by 28% (Selvin et al. 2004)and risk of intermittent claudication by 3.5- and 8.6-fold in men and women, respectively (Kannel and McGee 1985). DM may also lead to peripheral neuropathy and decreased resistance to infection, which increases the risk of infected foot ulcers. Patients with DM are at a higher risk of amputation and have reduced primary patency after revascularization as compared to non-diabetics (Bild et al. 1989; DeRubertis et al. 2008). The UKPDS study showed that the overall microvascular complication rate decreased by 25% by lowering blood glucose levels in type 2 diabetes with intensive therapy, which achieved a median HbA_{1c} of 7.0% compared with conventional therapy with a median HbA_{1c} of 7.9%. No significant effect on cardiovascular complications was observed. A non-significant ($p = 0.052$) 16% reduction in the risk of combined fatal or nonfatal myocardial infarction and sudden death was observed (UKPDS 1998).

The American Diabetic Association recommends maintaining hemoglobin A1c below 7% to reduce microvascular events (ADA 2010). This recommendation is endorsed by all three PAD guidelines. The ADA also recommends comprehensive foot care including proper footwear, regular podiatric foot and nail care, daily foot inspection, skin cleansing, and use of topical moisturizing creams (ADA 2010).

11.1.3 Dyslipidemia

The Heart Protection Study (HPS) randomized 20,536 high-risk patients to 40 mg/d of simvastatin or placebo, including 6,748 patients with PAD. PAD patients taking statins had a 25% cardiovascular risk reduction at 5 years independent of baseline LDL level (HPS 2002). Statin use is also associated with reduction in the risk of new or worsening claudication (Pedersen, Kjekshus et al. 1998). A RCT comparing high dose atorvastatin (80 mg) vs. placebo irrespective of baseline LDL cholesterol showed that high dose atorvastatin improves pain-free walking distance and community-based physical activity in patients with intermittent claudication, however there was no change noted in the maximal walking time. This beneficial effect was noted over statins cardiovascular risk reduction benefits. (Mohler, Hiatt et al. 2003).

The AHA / ACC and TASC 2 guidelines recommend the following for dyslipidemia management in patients with PAD (Dormandy and Rutherford 2000; Smith et al. 2001; Hirsch et al. 2006; Norgren, Hiatt et al. 2007).

- All patients should have low-density lipoprotein (LDL)- cholesterol <2.59 mmol/L (<100 mg/dL).
- In patients with PAD and a history of vascular disease in other beds (e.g. coronary artery disease) it is reasonable to lower LDL cholesterol levels to <1.81 mmol/L (<70 mg/dL).
- In patients with elevated triglyceride levels where the LDL cannot be accurately calculated, the LDL level should be directly measured and treated to the above targets. Alternatively, the non-HDL (high-density lipoprotein) cholesterol level can be calculated with a goal of <3.36 mmol/L (<130 mg/dL), and in high risk patients <2.59 mmol/L (<100 mg/Dl).
- Dietary modification should be the initial intervention to control abnormal lipid levels [B].

- In symptomatic PAD patients, statins should be the primary agents to lower LDL cholesterol levels to reduce the risk of cardiovascular events [A].

The SIGN guidelines recommend statins for patients with PAD and total cholesterol level > 3.5 mmol/l (63 mg/dl) (Network 2006).

The ACC/AHA and TASC II guidelines also recommended considering niacin / fibrates for raising HDL cholesterol and lowering triglycerides in patients with PAD who have abnormalities in these lipid fractions. Recently, the randomized trial, AIM - HIGH, failed to reduce the incidence of cardiovascular events among patients with CAD at 3 years and was terminated prematurely, raising questions about the benefit of niacin in patients with atherosclerotic vascular disease (http://www.aimhigh-heart.com/ 2011).

11.1.4 Management of hypertension

Blood pressure lowering by any pharmacological means reduces cardiovascular risk (Chobanian et al. 2003); however angiotensin converting enzyme inhibitors (ACEI) have benefit in patients with PAD beyond their effect on lowering blood pressure. The Heart Outcomes Prevention Evaluation (HOPE) study showed a 22% reduction in risk of MI, stroke, or vascular death in patients randomized to ramipril compared to placebo, independent of the blood pressure-lowering effect (Yusuf et al. 2000). Although once thought to worsen claudication, the safety of beta blockers, has been demonstrated in a meta-analysis of 11 trials of patients with PAD (Radack and Deck 1991); these agents are of benefit of patients with CAD, particularly among those with a history of prior myocardial infarction.

11.1.5 Anti-platelet therapy

11.1.5.1 Aspirin

Aspirin was initially recommended mainly based on a sub-group analysis of a Antithrombotic Trialists' Collaboration meta-analysis which is a meta-analysis of 42 RCT's published in 2002 which showed that anti-platelet therapy (primarily aspirin) reduced cardiovascular events by 23% in patients with symptomatic PAD including patients with IC (23%), those with peripheral grafts (22%) and those undergoing peripheral angioplasty (29%) (2002). However, this study had a lot of heterogeneity in selection criteria and different antiplatelet drugs used at different doses. Also the benefit of aspirin in asymptomatic PAD wasn't in this meta-analysis. A more recent meta-analysis of 18 RCT's including 5,269 patients with PAD, aspirin therapy alone or in combination with dipyridamole led to a non-significant 12% reduction in the primary end point of cardiovascular events(Berger et al. 2009). Two large RCT evaluated the benefit of aspirin in patients with asymptomatic PAD and found no benefit (Belch et al. 2008; Fowkes et al. 2010). However, both of these RCT's had populations with asymptomatic PAD with very mild decrease in ABI and characterized as mild PAD in general. In the Prevention of Progression of Arterial Disease and Diabetes (POPADAD) trial enrolled patients with ABI <0.99 and the Aspirin for Asymptomatic Atherosclerosis trial enrolled patient with ABI ≤0.95 which calculated by using the lower pedal pressure at the ankle. In standard clinical practice and guidelines, ABI is calculated using the higher pedal pressure (Belch et al. 2008; Fowkes et al. 2010). Hence, both of these studies had significant limitations in design and enrollment and no change in recommendation regarding anti-platelet therapy in this cohort have occurred (Belch et al. 2008; Fowkes et al. 2010).

11.1.5.2 Clopidogrel

In a post hoc subgroup analysis of 6,452 PAD patients in The Clopidogrel versus Aspirin in Patients at Risk of Ischemic Events (CAPRIE) trial, the incidence of stroke, MI, or vascular death was reduced by 24% among those randomized to clopidogrel compared to aspirin monotherapy (1996).

Dual antiplatelets therapy (DAPT) with aspirin and clopidogrel was not more effective than aspirin monotherapy in the Clopidogrel for High Atherothrombotic Risk and Ischemia Stabilization, Management and Avoidance (CHARISMA) study (Bhatt et al. 2006). However, post hoc analysis of the CHARISMA study revealed that DAPT was superior to aspirin monotherapy among patients with known symptomatic PAD at the time of enrollment (Bhatt et al. 2007). The combination of antiplatelet and anticoagulant therapy was evaluated in The Warfarin Anti-platelet Vascular Evaluation (WAVE) trial. This study found no incremental benefit of vitamin K antagonists when added to anti-platelet therapy for the prevention of cardiovascular events in patients with PAD (Anand et al. 2007). In fact, patients randomized to the combination of antiplatelet and anticoagulant therapy had an increase in life-threatening bleeding when compared with those randomized to anti-platelet therapy alone.

In general, all three PAD guidelines recommend antiplatelet therapy for PAD patients. Selection of an antiplatelet regimen (aspirin or clopidogrel or both or other antiplatelet medications) for the PAD patient should be individualized on the basis of tolerance and other clinical characteristics (i.e., bleeding risk) along with cost and guidance from regulatory agencies. (Dormandy and Rutherford 2000; Hirsch et al. 2006; Network 2006; Rooke et al. 2011). ACC / AHA guidelines strongly recommend antiplatelet therapy to reduce the risk of MI, stroke, and vascular death in individuals with symptomatic atherosclerotic lower extremity PAD, including those with intermittent claudication or critical limb ischemia, prior lower extremity revascularization (endovascular or surgical), or prior amputation for lower extremity ischemia (class IA). They feel that antiplatelet therapy can be useful to reduce the risk of MI, stroke, or vascular death in asymptomatic individuals with an ABI less than or equal to 0.90 (Class IIa C), however do not strongly recommend it given lack of definite evidence of any benefit (Rooke et al. 2011).

11.2 Medical therapy for claudication

11.2.1 Supervised exercise program

Many patients with PAD have severely impaired functional capacity, which leads to decreased quality of life (McDermott et al. 2004). A meta-analysis of 21 studies showed that patients with IC who underwent exercise training improved mean walking time by 180% and maximal walking time by 120% (Gardner and Poehlman 1995). Supervised treadmill exercises programs are also are more effective than lower extremity resistance training (McDermott et al. 2009). However, due to lack of reimbursement access to this important therapeutic intervention has been limited. In a Cochrane review of 8 RCT's evaluating supervised and unsupervised exercise among 319 participants with IC, statistically significant and clinically relevant improvements in maximal treadmill walking distance occurred with supervised compared with non-supervised exercise therapy during 12 weeks to 12 months of follow up (Bendermacher et al. 2006). Unsupervised therapy may be less effective than supervised therapy due to lack of motivation, compliance with recommended exercise, lack of progression of workload in the absence of professional supervision and concern for personal safety to advance the moderate claudication discomfort severity.

11.2.2 Pharmacological agents

Cilastozol is an FDA-approved medication for the management of IC. It is a reversible phosphodiesterase inhibitor whose exact mechanism of benefit is unclear. It inhibits platelet aggregation, thrombin formation, and vascular smooth muscle proliferation and acts as a vasodilator. It also increases HDL and lowers TG levels. In an analysis of 9 RCT's of cilastazol at dose of 100 mg BID, cilostazol showed a 50.7% improvement from baseline maximal walking distance compared to placebo (24.3%) (Pande et al. 2010). A Cochrane review found similar benefit (Robless et al. 2008). Given the increased incidence of sudden cardiac death with other phosphodiesterase inhibitors (e.g., milrinone), cilostazol is contraindicated in patients with heart failure and/ or ejection fraction less than 40% (Packer et al. 1991). The ACC/AHA guidelines have given cilostazol a grade IA recommendation for patients with intermittent claudication in the absence of heart failure.

Pentoxifylline is a methylxanthine derivative that decreases blood viscosity and has hemorheologic (improves erythrocyte and leukocyte deformability), anti-inflammatory, and antiproliferative effects. Its anti-claudication effect has been inconsistent. A study randomizing 698 patients with IC to cilostazol, pentoxifylline or placebo did not observe any difference between pentoxifylline and placebo (Dawson et al. 2000). ACC/AHA guidelines recommend using pentoxifylline as an alternative in patients who cannot tolerate cilostazol or in whom cilostazol is contraindicated.

11.2.3 Revascularization

Revascularization is only appropriate for symptomatic patients and should not be undertaken as prophylactic therapy for an asymptomatic limb (Hirsch et al. 2006). Revascularization is indicated in patients' with acute limb ischemia (ALI), CLI and among those with lifestyle- or vocation-limiting claudication who have failed a trial of medical therapy or who have highly favorable anatomy for endovascular therapy such as focal aorto-iliac disease (Hirsch et al. 2006) . Data comparing medical therapy with either endovascular or surgical therapy are scant. The ongoing Claudication: exercise vs endoluminal revascularization (CLEVER) trial is comparing medical therapy alone vs. medical therapy + supervised exercise vs. medical therapy + endovascular therapy (Murphy et al. 2008).

Endovascular therapy is currently the preferred mode of revascularization in cases where anatomy is more favorable (e.g., aorto-iliac disease). Endovascular therapy is less invasive, is associated with fewer complications and with shorter hospital stay as compared to bypass procedures. The durability of endovascular or surgical procedures depends on a number of factors including anatomic location (aorto-iliac revascularization whether open surgical or endovascular has superior long term outcomes compared with infra-inguinal revascularization), lesion characteristics, technical features (e.g., angioplasty alone vs. angioplasty + stent, type of surgical conduit used for surgical bypass). Hybrid procedures are performed for multi-level in an effort to minimize the overall operative risk of the revascularization (e.g., iliac artery stenting followed by femoral-popliteal bypass). Open surgical revascularization (e.g., bypass or endarterectomy) is typically reserved for endovascular failures or anatomy not likely to respond to an endovascular attempt.

12. Summary of the guideline recommendations for PAD

In table 4 we outline the grade A level of recommendation for PAD by TASC II guidelines. In table 5 we outline the class I recommendations by American College of Cardiology and American Heart association for PAD. Finally in table 6 we outline the differences in recommendations between the TASC II and American College of Cardiology / American Heart association guidelines for management of PAD.

TASC II grade A level of recommendation for peripheral arterial disease
All patients who smoke should receive a program of physician advice, group counseling sessions and nicotine replacement
Cessation rates can be enhanced by the addition of antidepressant drug therapy (bupropion) and nicotine replacement
All symptomatic PAD patients should have their LDL-cholesterol lowered to <2.59 mmol/L (<100 mg/dL)
In symptomatic PAD patients, statins should be the primary agents to lower LDL cholesterol levels to reduce the risk of cardiovascular events
All patients with hypertension should have blood pressure controlled to <140/90 mm Hg or <130/80 mm Hg if they also have diabetes or renal insufficiency
The Joint National Committee (JNC VII) and European guidelines for the management of hypertension in PAD should be followed
Beta-adrenergic blocking drugs are not contraindicated in PAD
All symptomatic patients with or without a history of other cardiovascular disease should be prescribed an antiplatelet drug long-term to reduce the risk of cardiovascular morbidity and mortality
Aspirin/ASA is effective in patients with PAD who also have clinical evidence of other forms of cardiovascular disease (coronary or carotid)
Routine coronary revascularization in preparation for vascular surgery is not recommended
When there are no contraindications, beta-adrenergic blockers should be given perioperatively to patients with peripheral artery disease undergoing vascular surgery in order to decrease cardiac morbidity and mortality
Supervised exercise should be made available as part of the initial treatment for all patients with peripheral artery disease
The most effective programs employ treadmill or track walking that is of sufficient intensity to bring on claudication, followed by rest, over the course of a 30–60 minute session. Exercise sessions are typically conducted three times a week for 3 months
A 3- to 6-month course of cilostazol should be first-line pharmacotherapy for the relief of claudication symptoms, as evidence shows both an improvement in treadmill exercise performance and in quality of life
Naftidrofuryl (Not available in United States of America) can also be considered for treatment of claudication symptoms
CLI patients should have aggressive modification of their cardiovascular risk factors
Antiplatelet therapy should be started preoperatively and continued as adjuvant pharmacotherapy after an endovascular or surgical procedure. Unless subsequently contraindicated, this should be continued indefinitely

Table 4. This table outlines TASC II grade A level of recommendation for peripheral arterial disease

Certain Class I recommendations for the Identification and Management of Peripheral artery Disease (PAD) by American Heart Association and American College of Cardiology with level of evidence (LOE)

All Patients with Peripheral Arterial Disease:

1. Smoking cessation, lipid lowering, and diabetes and hypertension treatment according to current national treatment guidelines are recommended for individuals with lower extremity peripheral arterial disease. (LOE: B)
2. -Blockers are effective antihypertensive agents and are not contraindicated in patients with PAD (LOE - A)
3. All Diabetic patients with PAD should properly care for their feet, and all skin lesions and ulcerations should be urgently addressed (LOE - B)
4. For patients who smoke, comprehensive smoking cessation, including behavior modification therapy, nicotine replacement, and/or bupropion should be strongly encouraged (LOE - B)
5. All patients with PAD should be treated with statins to achieve target LDL ≤ 100 mg/dl (LOE–B)
6. Antiplatelet therapy is indicated to reduce the risk of MI, stroke, and vascular death in individuals with symptomatic atherosclerotic lower extremity PAD, including those with intermittent claudication or critical limb ischemia, prior lower extremity revascularization or prior amputation for lower extremity ischemia (LOE:A)

Asymptomatic patients:

1. A history of walking impairment, claudication, ischemic rest pain, and/or nonhealing wounds is recommended as a required component of a standard ROS for adults 50 years and older who have atherosclerosis risk factors and for adults 65 years and older. (LOE: C)
2. Individuals with asymptomatic lower extremity peripheral arterial disease should be identified by examination and/or measurement of the ABI so that therapeutic interventions known to diminish their increased risk of MI, stroke, and death may be offered. (LOE: B)
3. Antiplatelet therapy is indicated for individuals with asymptomatic lower extremity peripheral arterial disease to reduce the risk of adverse cardiovascular ischemic events. (LOE: C)

Patients with intermittent claudication:

1. Patients should undergo a vascular physical examination, including measurement of the ABI. *(LOE: B)*
2. ABI should be measured after exercise if the resting index is normal. *(LOE: B)*
3. Patients should have significant functional impairment with a reasonable likelihood of symptomatic improvement and absence of other disease that would comparably limit exercise even if the claudication was improved before undergoing an evaluation for revascularization. *(LOE: C)*
4. Patients should be offered the option of endovascular or surgical therapies should: (a) be provided information regarding supervised claudication exercise therapy and pharmacotherapy; (b) receive comprehensive risk factor modification and antiplatelet therapy; (c) have a significant disability, either being unable to perform normal work or having serious impairment of other activities important to the patient; and (d) have lower extremity peripheral arterial disease lesion anatomy such that the revascularization procedure would have low risk and a high probability of initial and long-term success. *(LOE: C)*

Critical Limb Ischemia:

1. Patients should undergo expedited evaluation and treatment of factors that are known to increase the risk of amputation. (LOE: C)
2. Patients in whom open surgical repair is anticipated should undergo assessment of cardiovascular risk. (LOE: B)
3. Patients with a prior history of CLI or who have undergone successful treatment for CLI should be evaluated at least twice annually by a vascular specialist owing to the relatively high incidence of recurrence. (LOE: C)
4. Patients at risk of CLI should undergo regular inspection of the feet. (LOE: B)
5. Patients should be evaluated for aneurysmal disease. (LOE: B)
6. Systemic antibiotics should be initiated promptly in patients with CLI, skin ulcerations, and evidence of limb infection. (LOE: B)
7. Patients with CLI and skin breakdown should be referred to healthcare providers with specialized expertise in wound care. (LOE: B)
8. Patients who develop acute limb symptoms represent potential vascular emergencies and should be assessed immediately and treated by a specialist competent in treating vascular disease. (LOE: C)
9. Patients should receive verbal and written instructions regarding self-surveillance for potential recurrence. (LOE: C)

Acute Limb Ischemia:

Patients with acute limb ischemia and a salvageable extremity should undergo an emergent evaluation that defines the anatomic level of occlusion and that leads to prompt endovascular or surgical revascularization. *(LOE: B)*

Table 5. This table outlines Class I recommendations for the Identification and Management of Peripheral artery Disease (PAD) by American Heart Association and American College of Cardiology with level of evidence (LOE)

Comparison of ACC/AHA and TASC II guidelines
Evidence grading systems: Both the ACC/AHA and the TASC II guidelines utilize the ABC system of recommendation grading. The ACC/AHA guidelines provide further information by using an additional classification (Class I, II, IIa,IIb and III) for each of the examined procedures/treatments.
Diabetes therapy: Both guidelines suggest aggressive control of glycosylated hemoglobin (HbA_{1c}) in patients with diabetes to a target of <7.0%. Additionally, the TASC II guidelines indicate that, optimally, HbA_{1c} should be as close to 6% as possible.
Claudication: The guidelines recommend different agents as second-line alternatives to cilostazol in patients with claudication - the ACC/AHA recommends pentoxyfylline and the TASC II guidelines recommend naftidrofuryl (not available in USA).
Hypertension: The ACC/AHA guidelines provide no indication as to the initial pharmacotherapeutic strategy to be utilized as antihypertensive medication in patients with PAD. In contrast, the TASC II guidelines advocate the use of either thiazide diuretics or angiotensin-converting enzyme (ACE) inhibitors as first-line blood pressure lowering therapy.
Lipid-lowering therapy: The TASC II guidelines recommend that the initial strategy for reducing lipid levels should focus on the use of dietary modifications whilst the ACC/AHA guidelines recommend the use of statins as first-line therapy for lipid level reduction.
In summary, there is little difference between the guidelines in terms of recommendations for clinical practice (Mohler and Giri 2008)

Table 6. This table outlines the main differences between the ACC/AHA PAD guidelines and TASC II guidelines are summarized in this table

13. Conclusions

PAD is a common disease, present in more than 8 million Americans and is associated with a relatively high risk of cardiovascular events. Nevertheless, it remains under-recognized by healthcare providers and patients alike. Increased awareness, earlier identification of the disease and aggressive medical therapy and vascular risk factor modification would reduce the likelihood of fatal and non-fatal cardiovascular events and improve overall functional status and quality of life.

14. References

(1996). "A randomised, blinded, trial of clopidogrel versus aspirin in patients at risk of ischaemic events (CAPRIE). CAPRIE Steering Committee." *Lancet* 348(9038): 1329-1339.

(2002). "Collaborative meta-analysis of randomised trials of antiplatelet therapy for prevention of death, myocardial infarction, and stroke in high risk patients." *BMJ* 324(7329): 71-86.

(2003). "Peripheral arterial disease in people with diabetes." *Diabetes care* 26(12): 3333-3341.

Aboyans, V., M. H. Criqui, et al. (2006). "Risk factors for progression of peripheral arterial disease in large and small vessels." *Circulation* 113(22): 2623-2629.

ADA (2010). "Standards of medical care in diabetes--2010." *Diabetes care* 33 Suppl 1: S11-61.

Allison, M. A. et al. (2007). "Ethnic-specific prevalence of peripheral arterial disease in the United States." *American journal of preventive medicine* 32(4): 328-333.

Anand, S. et al. (2007). "Oral anticoagulant and antiplatelet therapy and peripheral arterial disease." *The New England journal of medicine* 357(3): 217-227.

Anthonisen, N. R. et al. (2005). "The effects of a smoking cessation intervention on 14.5-year mortality: a randomized clinical trial." *Annals of internal medicine* 142(4): 233-239.

Aronow, W. S. et al. (2002). "Prevalence and incidence of cardiovascular disease in 1160 older men and 2464 older women in a long-term health care facility." *The journals of gerontology. Series A, Biological sciences and medical sciences* 57(1): M45-46.

Beckman, J. A et al. (2002). "Diabetes and atherosclerosis: epidemiology, pathophysiology, and management." *JAMA* 287(19): 2570-2581.

Belch, J. et al. (2008). "The prevention of progression of arterial disease and diabetes (POPADAD) trial: factorial randomised placebo controlled trial of aspirin and antioxidants in patients with diabetes and asymptomatic peripheral arterial disease." *BMJ* 337: a1840.

Bendermacher, B. L. et al. (2006). "Supervised exercise therapy versus non-supervised exercise therapy for intermittent claudication." *Cochrane database of systematic reviews*(2): CD005263.

Berger, J. S. et al. (2009). "Aspirin for the prevention of cardiovascular events in patients with peripheral artery disease: a meta-analysis of randomized trials." *JAMA* 301(18): 1909-1919.

Bhatt, D. L. et al. (2007). "Patients with prior myocardial infarction, stroke, or symptomatic peripheral arterial disease in the CHARISMA trial." *Journal of the American College of Cardiology* 49(19): 1982-1988.

Bhatt, D. L. et al. (2006). "Clopidogrel and aspirin versus aspirin alone for the prevention of atherothrombotic events." *The New England journal of medicine* 354(16): 1706-1717.

Bild, D. E. et al. (1989). "Lower-extremity amputation in people with diabetes. Epidemiology and prevention." *Diabetes care* 12(1): 24-31.

Boushey, C. J. et al. (1995). "A quantitative assessment of plasma homocysteine as a risk factor for vascular disease. Probable benefits of increasing folic acid intakes." *JAMA* 274(13): 1049-1057.

Bowlin, S. J. et al. (1994). "Epidemiology of intermittent claudication in middle-aged men." *Am J Epidemiol* 140(5): 418-430.

Cheng, S. W. et al. (1999). "Screening for asymptomatic carotid stenosis in patients with peripheral vascular disease: a prospective study and risk factor analysis." *Cardiovasc Surg* 7(3): 303-309.

Chobanian, A. V. et al. (2003). "The Seventh Report of the Joint National Committee on Prevention, Detection, Evaluation, and Treatment of High Blood Pressure: the JNC 7 report." *JAMA* 289(19): 2560-2572.

Conlan, M. G. et al. (1993). "Associations of factor VIII and von Willebrand factor with age, race, sex, and risk factors for atherosclerosis. The Atherosclerosis Risk in Communities (ARIC) Study." *Thrombosis and haemostasis* 70(3): 380-385.

Criqui, M. H. et al. (1996). "The correlation between symptoms and non-invasive test results in patients referred for peripheral arterial disease testing." *Vascular medicine* 1(1): 65-71.

Criqui, M. H., et al. (1985). "The prevalence of peripheral arterial disease in a defined population." *Circulation* 71(3): 510-515.

Criqui, M. H. et al. (1992). "Mortality over a period of 10 years in patients with peripheral arterial disease." *The New England journal of medicine* 326(6): 381-386.

Critchley, J. and S. Capewell (2004). "Smoking cessation for the secondary prevention of coronary heart disease." *Cochrane database of systematic reviews*(1): CD003041.

Darling, R. C. et al. (1972). "Quantitative segmental pulse volume recorder: a clinical tool." *Surgery* 72(6): 873-877.

Dawson, D. L. et al. (2000). "A comparison of cilostazol and pentoxifylline for treating intermittent claudication." *The American journal of medicine* 109(7): 523-530.

DeRubertis, B. G. et al. (2008). "Reduced primary patency rate in diabetic patients after percutaneous intervention results from more frequent presentation with limb-threatening ischemia." *Journal of vascular surgery* 47(1): 101-108.

Diehm, C. et al. (2009). "Mortality and vascular morbidity in older adults with asymptomatic versus symptomatic peripheral artery disease." *Circulation* 120(21): 2053-2061.

Dormandy, J. A. and R. B. Rutherford (2000). "Management of peripheral arterial disease (PAD). TASC Working Group. TransAtlantic Inter-Society Consensus (TASC)." *Journal of vascular surgery* 31(1 Pt 2): S1-S296.

Folsom, A. R. et al. (1992). "Distributions of hemostatic variables in blacks and whites: population reference values from the Atherosclerosis Risk in Communities (ARIC) Study." *Ethnicity & disease* 2(1): 35-46.

Fowkes, F. G. (1988). "The measurement of atherosclerotic peripheral arterial disease in epidemiological surveys." *International journal of epidemiology* 17(2): 248-254.

Fowkes, F. et al. (1992). "Smoking, lipids, glucose intolerance, and blood pressure as risk factors for peripheral atherosclerosis compared with ischemic heart disease in the Edinburgh Artery Study." *American journal of epidemiology* 135(4): 331-340.

Fowkes, F. G. et al. (2008). "Ankle brachial index combined with Framingham Risk Score to predict cardiovascular events and mortality: a meta-analysis." *JAMA* 300(2): 197-208.

Fowkes, F. G. et al. (2010). "Aspirin for prevention of cardiovascular events in a general population screened for a low ankle brachial index: a randomized controlled trial." *JAMA* 303(9): 841-848.

Gardner, A. W. and E. T. Poehlman (1995). "Exercise rehabilitation programs for the treatment of claudication pain. A meta-analysis." *JAMA* 274(12): 975-980.

Gerhard, G. T. et al. (1999). "Higher total homocysteine concentrations and lower folate concentrations in premenopausal black women than in premenopausal white women." *The American journal of clinical nutrition* 70(2): 252-260.

Hajjar, K. A. (1993). "Homocysteine-induced modulation of tissue plasminogen activator binding to its endothelial cell membrane receptor." *J Clin Invest* 91(6): 2873-2879.

Hertzer, N. R. et al. (1984). "Coronary artery disease in peripheral vascular patients. A classification of 1000 coronary angiograms and results of surgical management." *Annals of surgery* 199(2): 223-233.

Hiatt, W. R. (2001). "Medical treatment of peripheral arterial disease and claudication." The *New England journal of medicine* 344(21): 1608-1621.

Hiatt, W. R. et al. (1995). "Effect of diagnostic criteria on the prevalence of peripheral arterial disease. The San Luis Valley Diabetes Study." *Circulation* 91(5): 1472-1479.

Hirsch, A. T. et al. (2001). "Peripheral arterial disease detection, awareness, and treatment in primary care." *JAMA* 286(11): 1317-1324.

Hirsch, A. T., Z. J. Haskal, et al. (2006). "ACC/AHA 2005 Practice Guidelines for the management of patients with peripheral arterial disease (lower extremity, renal, mesenteric, and abdominal aortic): a collaborative report from the American Association for Vascular Surgery/Society for Vascular Surgery, Society for Cardiovascular Angiography and Interventions, Society for Vascular Medicine and Biology, Society of Interventional Radiology, and the ACC/AHA Task Force on Practice Guidelines (Writing Committee to Develop Guidelines for the Management of Patients With Peripheral Arterial Disease): endorsed by the American Association of Cardiovascular and Pulmonary Rehabilitation; National Heart, Lung, and Blood Institute; Society for Vascular Nursing; TransAtlantic Inter-Society Consensus; and Vascular Disease Foundation." *Circulation* 113(11): e463-654.

HPS (2002). "MRC/BHF Heart Protection Study of cholesterol lowering with simvastatin in 20,536 high-risk individuals: a randomised placebo-controlled trial." *Lancet* 360(9326): 7-22.

http://www.aimhigh-heart.com/. (2011).

Ingolfsson, I. O. et al. (1994). "A marked decline in the prevalence and incidence of intermittent claudication in Icelandic men 1968-1986: a strong relationship to smoking and serum cholesterol--the Reykjavik Study." *Journal of clinical epidemiology* 47(11): 1237-1243.

Jorenby, D. E. et al. (2006). "Efficacy of varenicline, an alpha4beta2 nicotinic acetylcholine receptor partial agonist, vs placebo or sustained-release bupropion for smoking cessation: a randomized controlled trial." *JAMA* 296(1): 56-63.

Jorenby, D. E. et al. (1999). "A controlled trial of sustained-release bupropion, a nicotine patch, or both for smoking cessation." *The New England journal of medicine* 340(9): 685-691.

Jude, E. B. et al. (2001). "Peripheral arterial disease in diabetic and nondiabetic patients: a comparison of severity and outcome." *Diabetes care* 24(8): 1433-1437.

Kannel, W. B. and D. L. McGee (1985). "Update on some epidemiologic features of intermittent claudication: the Framingham Study." *Journal of the American Geriatrics Society* 33(1): 13-18.

Kannel, W. B. and D. Shurtleff (1973). "The Framingham Study. Cigarettes and the development of intermittent claudication." *Geriatrics* 28(2): 61-68.

Klop, R. B. et al. (1991). "Screening of the internal carotid arteries in patients with peripheral vascular disease by colour-flow duplex scanning." *European journal of vascular surgery* 5(1): 41-45.

Law, M. and J. L. Tang (1995). "An analysis of the effectiveness of interventions intended to help people stop smoking." *Archives of internal medicine* 155(18): 1933-1941.

Leng, G. C. and F. G. Fowkes (1992). "The Edinburgh Claudication Questionnaire: an improved version of the WHO/Rose Questionnaire for use in epidemiological surveys." *Journal of clinical epidemiology* 45(10): 1101-1109.

Lijmer, J. G. et al. (1996). "ROC analysis of noninvasive tests for peripheral arterial disease." *Ultrasound in medicine & biology* 22(4): 391-398.

Marso, S. P. and W. R. Hiatt (2006). "Peripheral arterial disease in patients with diabetes." *Journal of the American College of Cardiology* 47(5): 921-929.

McDermott, M. et al. (2009). "Treadmill exercise and resistance training in patients with peripheral arterial disease with and without intermittent claudication: a randomized controlled trial." *JAMA* 301(2): 165-174.

McDermott, M. M. et al. (2002). "The ankle brachial index is associated with leg function and physical activity: the Walking and Leg Circulation Study." *Annals of internal medicine* 136(12): 873-883.

McDermott, M. M. et al. (2004). "Functional decline in peripheral arterial disease: associations with the ankle brachial index and leg symptoms." *JAMA* 292(4): 453-461.

McFalls, E. O. et al. (2004). "Coronary-artery revascularization before elective major vascular surgery." *The New England journal of medicine* 351(27): 2795-2804.

Meijer, W. T. et al. (1998). "Peripheral arterial disease in the elderly: The Rotterdam Study." *Arterioscler Thromb Vasc Biol* 18(2): 185-192.

Mohler, E., 3rd and J. Giri (2008). "Management of peripheral arterial disease patients: comparing the ACC/AHA and TASC-II guidelines." *Current medical research and opinion* 24(9): 2509-2522.

Mohler, E. R., 3rd, W. R. Hiatt, et al. (2003). "Cholesterol reduction with atorvastatin improves walking distance in patients with peripheral arterial disease." *Circulation* 108(12): 1481-1486.

Murabito, J. M. et al. (1997). "Intermittent claudication. A risk profile from The Framingham Heart Study." *Circulation* 96(1): 44-49.

Murabito, J. M et al. (2002). "Prevalence and clinical correlates of peripheral arterial disease in the Framingham Offspring Study." *American heart journal* 143(6): 961-965.

Murphy, T. P. et al. (2008). "The Claudication: Exercise Vs. Endoluminal Revascularization (CLEVER) study: rationale and methods." *Journal of vascular surgery* 47(6): 1356-1363.

Ness, J. et al. (2000). "Risk factors for symptomatic peripheral arterial disease in older persons in an academic hospital-based geriatrics practice." *Journal of the American Geriatrics Society* 48(3): 312-314.

Network, S. I. G. (2006). "Diagnosis and management of peripheral arterial disease: a national clinical guideline." Edinburgh, Scotland: *SIGN.*

Norgren, L. et al. (2007). "Inter-Society Consensus for the Management of Peripheral Arterial Disease (TASC II)." *Journal of vascular surgery* 45 Suppl S: S5-67.

O'Hare, A. M. et al. (2003). "Impact of renal insufficiency on short-term morbidity and mortality after lower extremity revascularization: data from the Department of Veterans Affairs' National Surgical Quality Improvement Program." *Journal of the American Society of Nephrology : JASN* 14(5): 1287-1295.

O'Hare, A. M. et al. (2004). "High prevalence of peripheral arterial disease in persons with renal insufficiency: results from the National Health and Nutrition Examination Survey 1999-2000." *Circulation* 109(3): 320-323.

Ostchega, Y., et al. (2007). "Prevalence of peripheral arterial disease and risk factors in persons aged 60 and older: data from the National Health and Nutrition Examination Survey 1999-2004." *Journal of the American Geriatrics Society* 55(4): 583-589.

Packer, M. et al. (1991). "Effect of oral milrinone on mortality in severe chronic heart failure. The PROMISE Study Research Group." *The New England journal of medicine* 325(21): 1468-1475.

Pande, R. L et al. (2010). "A pooled analysis of the durability and predictors of treatment response of cilostazol in patients with intermittent claudication." *Vascular medicine* 15(3): 181-188.

Pedersen et al. (1998). "Effect of simvastatin on ischemic signs and symptoms in the Scandinavian simvastatin survival study (4S)." *The American journal of cardiology* 81(3): 333-335.

Radack, K. and C. Deck (1991). "Beta-adrenergic blocker therapy does not worsen intermittent claudication in subjects with peripheral arterial disease. A meta-analysis of randomized controlled trials." *Archives of internal medicine* 151(9): 1769-1776.

Rigotti, N. A. et al. (2010). "Efficacy and safety of varenicline for smoking cessation in patients with cardiovascular disease: a randomized trial." *Circulation* 121(2): 221-229.

Robless, P. et al. (2008). "Cilostazol for peripheral arterial disease." *Cochrane database of systematic reviews*(1): CD003748.

Rooke, T. W. et al. (2011). "2011 ACCF/AHA Focused Update of the Guideline for the Management of Patients With Peripheral Artery Disease (Updating the 2005 Guideline): A Report of the American College of Cardiology Foundation/American Heart Association Task Force on Practice Guidelines." *Circulation.*

Rose, G. A. (1962). "The diagnosis of ischaemic heart pain and intermittent claudication in field surveys." *Bull World Health Organ* 27: 645-658.

Sapoval, M. R. et al. (1996). "Self-expandable stents for the treatment of iliac artery obstructive lesions: long-term success and prognostic factors." *AJR Am J Roentgenol* 166(5): 1173-1179.

Selvin, E. and T. P. Erlinger (2004). "Prevalence of and risk factors for peripheral arterial disease in the United States: results from the National Health and Nutrition Examination Survey, 1999-2000." *Circulation* 110(6): 738-743.

Selvin, E. et al. (2004). "Meta-analysis: glycosylated hemoglobin and cardiovascular disease in diabetes mellitus." *Annals of internal medicine* 141(6): 421-431.

Shammas, N. W. et al. (2003). "In-hospital complications of peripheral vascular interventions using unfractionated heparin as the primary anticoagulant." The *Journal of invasive cardiology* 15(5): 242-246.

Sikkink, C. J. et al. (1997). "Decreased ankle/brachial indices in relation to morbidity and mortality in patients with peripheral arterial disease." *Vascular medicine* 2(3): 169-173.

Smith, G. D. et al. (1990). "Intermittent claudication, heart disease risk factors, and mortality. The Whitehall Study." *Circulation* 82(6): 1925-1931.

Smith, S. C., et al. (2001). "AHA/ACC Scientific Statement: AHA/ACC guidelines for preventing heart attack and death in patients with atherosclerotic cardiovascular disease: 2001 update: A statement for healthcare professionals from the American Heart Association and the American College of Cardiology." *Circulation* 104(13): 1577-1579.

Spertus, J., et al. (2004). "The peripheral artery questionnaire: a new disease-specific health status measure for patients with peripheral arterial disease." *American heart journal* 147(2): 301-308.

Steg, P. G. et al. (2007). "One-year cardiovascular event rates in outpatients with atherothrombosis." *JAMA* 297(11): 1197-1206.

Symes, J. F. et al. (1984). "Doppler waveform analysis versus segmental pressure and pulse-volume recording: assessment of occlusive disease in the lower extremity." *Canadian journal of surgery. Journal canadien de chirurgie* 27(4): 345-347.

Tonstad, S. et al. (2003). "Bupropion SR for smoking cessation in smokers with cardiovascular disease: a multicentre, randomised study." *European heart journal* 24(10): 946-955.

UKPDS (1998). "Intensive blood-glucose control with sulphonylureas or insulin compared with conventional treatment and risk of complications in patients with type 2 diabetes (UKPDS 33). UK Prospective Diabetes Study (UKPDS) Group." *Lancet* 352(9131): 837-853.

Valentine, R. J. et al. (1994). "Coronary artery disease is highly prevalent among patients with premature peripheral vascular disease." *Journal of vascular surgery* 19(4): 668-674.

Vidula, H. et al. (2008). "Biomarkers of inflammation and thrombosis as predictors of near-term mortality in patients with peripheral arterial disease: a cohort study." *Annals of internal medicine* 148(2): 85-93.

Wattanakit, K. et al. (2005). "Risk factors for peripheral arterial disease incidence in persons with diabetes: the Atherosclerosis Risk in Communities (ARIC) Study." *Atherosclerosis* 180(2): 389-397.

Willigendael, E. M. et al. (2005). "Smoking and the patency of lower extremity bypass grafts: a meta-analysis." *Journal of vascular surgery* 42(1): 67-74.

Yusuf, S., P. Sleight, et al. (2000). "Effects of an angiotensin-converting-enzyme inhibitor, ramipril, on cardiovascular events in high-risk patients. The Heart Outcomes Prevention Evaluation Study Investigators." *The New England journal of medicine* 342(3): 145-153.